# The Smoking Paradox

# The Smoking Paradox

UNFILTERED TRUTHS

Ehsan Sheroy

Kellie D. Sikora

# Contents

| | |
|---|---|
| INDEX | 1 |
| Introduction | 3 |
| Chapter 1 | 6 |
| Chapter 2 | 25 |
| Chapter 3 | 38 |
| Chapter 4 | 54 |
| Chapter 5 | 67 |
| Chapter 6 | 82 |
| Chapter 7 | 98 |
| Chapter 8 | 112 |
| Chapter 9 | 128 |

# INDEX

**Introduction**

**Chapter 1: Up in Smoke**
1.1 Introduction to the pervasive nature of smoking in society
1.2 Statistics on global tobacco consumption
1.3 Overview of the health risks associated with smoking

**Chapter 2: Origins and Influence**
2.1 Historical background of tobacco use
2.2 Exploration of cultural and societal influences on smoking
2.3 The role of advertising and media in promoting smoking

**Chapter 3: The Addictive Puzzle**
3.1 Understanding the science behind nicotine addiction
3.2 Personal stories of addiction and attempts to quit
3.3 The psychological aspects of smoking and dependency

**Chapter 4: Smoke and Mirrors – The Tobacco Industry's Secrets**
4.1 Unveiling the tactics used by the tobacco industry
4.2 Exposé on marketing strategies targeting vulnerable populations
4.3 Legal battles and controversies surrounding the tobacco industry

**Chapter 5: The Health Toll**
5.1 In-depth exploration of smoking-related health issues
5.2 Personal testimonies of individuals affected by smoking-related diseases
5.3 Economic burden on healthcare systems due to smoking-related illnesses

**Chapter 6: Breaking the Chains – Quitting Challenges**
6.1 Analysis of various cessation methods
6.2 The psychological and physical hurdles of quitting

6.3 Success stories of individuals who successfully quit smoking

**Chapter 7: The Paradoxical Pleasure**
7.1 Examining the perceived pleasures of smoking
7.2 Cultural and social aspects of smoking as a social activity
7.3 The role of stress relief and relaxation in smoking behavior

**Chapter 8: Smoke Signals – Global Perspectives**
8.1 International variations in smoking prevalence
8.2 Government policies and anti-smoking initiatives around the world
8.3 Cultural attitudes towards smoking in different societies

**Chapter 9: Clearing the Air – The Path Forward**
9.1 Advocacy for tobacco control and public health policies
9.2 Innovative approaches to smoking cessation
9.3 The potential for a smoke-free future and the role of society in achieving it

# Introduction

The demonstration of smoking has been a social steady for quite a long time, woven into the texture of social orders around the world. It's an incomprehensible custom, one that has endured through moving standards and developing understandings of wellbeing. The Smoking Mystery typifies a mind boggling transaction of social, social, mental, and physiological elements that add to the persevering through allure of smoking, compared against a consistently developing collection of proof featuring its inconvenient wellbeing impacts.

From old ceremonies to the cutting edge cigarette, smoking has worn different veils, transforming to line up with the soul of various periods. The early ceremonies of tobacco use by native people groups were saturated with custom and otherworldly importance, with the smoke going about as a scaffold between the human and heavenly domains. This antiquated practice, notwithstanding, changed decisively with the appearance of Europeans in the Americas, prompting the commodification and worldwide spread of tobacco.

Quick forward to the industrialized twentieth 100 years, and smoking went through a critical change. Cigarettes, bundled in alluring plans, became inseparable from disobedience, marvelousness, and complexity. Hollywood symbols, frequently seen with a cigarette close by, added to the romanticization of smoking, establishing its spot in the social climate. The appeal of smoke rings and the musical dance of breathed out tufts became emblematic signals inseparably connected to thoughts of opportunity and self-articulation.

The mystery extends as science started disentangling the multifaceted connection among smoking and wellbeing. Epidemiological examinations enlightened the staggering wellbeing results of tobacco use, connecting it to a reiteration of sicknesses, from cellular breakdown in the lungs to cardiovascular problems. The Top health spokesperson's milestone report during the 1960s denoted a defining moment, setting off open mindfulness missions and hostile to smoking drives. States overall wrestled with the mystery of advancing general wellbeing while at the same time adjusting the monetary interests of strong tobacco ventures.

Regardless of mounting proof and general wellbeing efforts, the charm of smoking perseveres. The Smoking Mystery stretches out past the physiological dependence on nicotine; it digs into the mental and sociocultural aspects that support this apparently silly way of behaving. Smoking, for some, turns into a survival strategy, a custom implanted in snapshots of stress, festivity, or isolation. The demonstration of lighting a cigarette, breathing in profoundly, and breathing out leisurely turns into an instinctive encounter, a substantial anchor in the tumult of life.

Peer pressure, defiant undercurrents, and the craving for social acknowledgment assume significant parts in propagating the mystery. Smoking frequently becomes entwined with character, a marker of having a place with a specific subculture or gathering. The defiant charm of smoking appears in the rebellion of cultural standards, a signal that challenges authority and questions laid out ideal models. The picture of the solitary smoker, outlined against the night sky, addresses a longing for independence, even despite realized wellbeing gambles.

The Smoking Mystery additionally entwines with issues of financial dissimilarity. Smoking rates are in many cases higher in underestimated networks, where the burdens of destitution, restricted admittance to training, and an absence of medical services worsen the difficulties of stopping. The conundrum here lies in the way that the people who can least manage the cost of the wellbeing results of smoking are in many cases the ones most trapped in its web.

Innovative progressions delivered options like e-cigarettes, showcased as a more secure option in contrast to conventional smoking. However, the quickly developing scene of vaping and its own arrangement of wellbeing concerns add one more layer to the Catch 22. Are these choices truly a stage towards hurt decrease, or do they simply sustain the pattern of fixation under an alternate pretense?

Understanding the Smoking Mystery requires a multidisciplinary approach that winds around together history, social science, brain research, general wellbeing, and financial matters. It requests an investigation of the perplexing embroidered artwork of human way of behaving and the variables that shape our decisions, in any event, when confronted with overpowering proof of damage. The Unfiltered Bits of insight implanted in this conundrum challenge us to defy the physiological habit as well as the profoundly imbued social and mental elements that support smoking notwithstanding sane information.

This investigation into the Smoking Mystery welcomes us to scrutinize our presumptions, challenge cultural standards, and dive into the intricacies of human way of behaving. It prompts us to look at the job of publicizing, media, and social elements in sustaining a propensity that, on a judicious level, appears to be in conflict with the quest for prosperity. As we unwind the layers of this Catch 22, we are gone up against with moral contemplations encompassing individual decisions, industry impact, and public arrangement.

The Unfiltered Insights that arise force us to rethink our way to deal with smoking end, perceiving that a simply clinical or reformatory position might miss the mark in tending to the mind boggling trap of impacts that support the propensity. It coaxes us to investigate creative mediations that consider the mental and social elements of smoking, recognizing that a one-size-fits-all approach may not be viable in breaking the chains of enslavement.

The Smoking Mystery, at its center, welcomes a nuanced discussion about individual organization and cultural obligation. It prompts us to consider the strain between individual flexibilities and general wellbeing objectives, encouraging a fragile equilibrium that regards independence while defending the prosperity of networks. Disentangling this conundrum expects us to pay attention to the tales of smokers, to figure out the profoundly private reasons that tight spot them to this propensity, and to move toward the issue with sympathy and empathy.

In exploring the Smoking Catch 22, we are faced with the test of accommodating clashing stories - the defiant charm of smoke-filled dreams and the obvious, proof based real factors of wellbeing gambles. It welcomes us to contemplate the restrictions of individual flexibility in a world interconnected by shared spaces and aggregate prosperity. The Unfiltered Insights implanted in this Catch 22 propel us to rise above oversimplified divisions and embrace a more nuanced comprehension of human way of behaving, recognizing that the foundations of this conundrum stretch out a long ways past the limits of a cigarette pack.

As we leave on this investigation of the Smoking Oddity and its Unfiltered Bits of insight, we are called to ponder the intricacies of smoking as well as on the more extensive embroidery of human way of behaving and society. The oddity welcomes us to address, to participate in discourse, and to look for arrangements that resound with the unpredictable dance of values, convictions, and desires that characterize us as people and as a system. The excursion into the core of the Smoking Conundrum is an excursion into the profundities of human instinct, a mission for understanding that goes past the surface to uncover the significant insights that shape our decisions and our reality.

# Chapter 1

**Up in Smoke**

In the modest community of Crestwood, settled between moving slopes and immense territories of vegetation, life unfurled in an anticipated mood. The townsfolk approached their everyday schedules, willfully ignorant of the situation that was unobtrusively unfolding not too far off. Much to their dismay that their curious presence was going to be immersed in a storm of confusion and vulnerability.

Everything started on an apparently common Tuesday morning. The sun cast its warm beams over the languid town, and a delicate breeze stirred through the leaves of the old oaks that lined the roads. The residents tasted their espresso and traded merriments, totally unmindful of the series of situation that would before long develop.

As the clock struck early afternoon, a tuft of smoke rose on the edges of Crestwood. It surged high up like a dull sign, grabbing the eye of the residents who stopped in their tracks to look in bewilderment. Alarm started to fan out like quickly as bits of hearsay flowed about the wellspring of the inauspicious smoke.

The local group of fire-fighters raced to the scene, alarms howling somewhere far off. The once-peaceful town square currently hummed with restless murmurs as occupants accumulated to observe the unfurling show. Eyes extended and hearts beat as the firemen combat the blast, their hoses splashing water in a frantic endeavor to suppress the blazes.

The wellspring of the fire before long became evident — a rambling manufacturing plant that had been a foundation of Crestwood's economy for quite a long time. The Summit Assembling Plant, which had utilized ages of the town's occupants, was presently a bursting hellfire. Thick, dark smoke surged up high, creating a shaded area over the town's feeling of safety.

As the fire seethed on, the residents watched in dismay as their livelihoods disintegrated. The production line, when an image of success, presently remained as a singed skeleton against the background of the sunset. The harsh smell of consuming flotsam and jetsam waited in the air, a severe sign of the delicacy of their once-steady lives.

In the days that followed, Crestwood turned into a town in grieving. The deficiency of the Top Assembling Plant sent shockwaves through the local area, abandoning a void that no measure of compassion could fill. Families confronted vulnerability as providers secured themselves without positions, and the once-flourishing neighborhood economy started to disintegrate.

In the midst of the destruction, a gathering of concerned residents assembled to examine the eventual fate of Crestwood. The municipal events were full of strain as occupants wrestled with the overwhelming undertaking of remaking their lives. The inquiry at the forefront of everybody's thoughts was basic at this point significant: How does a local area come to life when all that they once realized has been diminished to rubble?

Amidst the mayhem, a charming pioneer rose up out of the shadows. Sarah Mitchell, a deep rooted inhabitant of Crestwood, ventured forward to energize her kindred residents. With an assurance that verged on hardheadedness, she pronounced that Crestwood wouldn't be characterized by the awfulness of the fire but instead by its capacity to come to life.

Sarah's revitalizing cry reverberated with the residents, and a feeling of solidarity started to flourish. Boards of trustees were framed to address the different difficulties confronting the local area — joblessness, lodging, and the general feeling of sadness that lingered over Crestwood like a foreboding shadow. It was an overwhelming undertaking, yet the aggregate soul of the residents ended up being an awe-inspiring phenomenon.

As the days transformed into weeks, Crestwood went through a change. The once-crushed town square turned into a center of action as volunteers worked resolutely to remake what had been lost. The sound of mallets and saws reverberated through the air as new designs miraculously rose like a phoenix after the old. It was a sluggish and exhausting interaction, however with each nail pounded into place, Crestwood recaptured a feeling of direction.

Amidst the reconstructing endeavors, an unforeseen partner arose. An adjoining town, propelled by Crestwood's strength, offered help as provisions, labor supply, and a feeling of fortitude. The motion was met with appreciation and modesty, as Crestwood understood that they were in good company in their battle. The fire that had taken steps to consume them had, in a bizarre bit of destiny, lighted a fire of solidarity that consumed more brilliant than any time in recent memory.

As the actual injuries of the fire started to mend, the profound scars waited. Numerous inhabitants wrestled with the injury of losing their positions as well as their feeling of safety. The once-affectionate local area thought of itself as broken, as people adapted to the fallout in their own particular manners. Some looked for comfort in treatment and care groups, while others drenched themselves in the reconstructing system as a type of therapy.

One especially impactful second came when a gathering of nearby craftsmen chose to channel their melancholy into a cooperative task. The scorched remaining parts of the Summit Assembling Plant turned into a material for a wall painting that portrayed the town's excursion from misery to trust. It was a visual portrayal of Crestwood's versatility, a demonstration of the dauntless soul of a local area that wouldn't be characterized by misfortune.

As the wall painting came to fruition, the residents accumulated to observe the change of a difficult update into an image of motivation. The once-stifled eyes of the industrial facility presently shimmered with lively varieties, recounting an account of misfortune, constancy, and, eventually, recharging. It filled in as a strong update that even despite difficulty, excellence could rise up out of the cinders.

The revamping system likewise provoked a reconsideration of Crestwood's financial establishment. The deficiency of the Top Assembling Plant constrained the local area to investigate new roads of development and supportability. Neighborhood business visionaries immediately jumping all over the chance to begin independent companies, infusing a feeling of imperativeness into the town's economy.

Crestwood turned into a sanctuary for inventiveness and development, with craftsmans, experts, and tech new companies finding a home in the midst of the remade structures. The town's personality moved from a modern center point to a different and dynamic local area that embraced change. The scars of the fire became symbols of honor, worn proudly by a town that had endured the hardship and arisen more grounded on the opposite side.

Amidst Crestwood's change, Sarah Mitchell kept on assuming a significant part. Her initiative style, portrayed by compassion and versatility, acquired her the trust and deference of the residents. As the chosen city hall leader, she worked energetically to explore the intricacies of remaking, tending to the different necessities of the local area with a consistent hand.

Sarah's vision reached out past the actual reproduction of Crestwood. She perceived the significance of recuperating the profound injuries that waited underneath the surface. Emotional well-being drives, directing administrations, and local area occasions became essential parts of Crestwood's recuperation plan. The town's process was tied in with modifying structures as well as about supporting the prosperity of its occupants.

Amidst Crestwood's resurrection, a feeling of satisfaction saturated the air. The residents thought back on the fire not as a misfortune that characterized them but rather as an impetus for positive change. The scars on the scene filled in as a steady sign of the flexibility that coursed through their veins. Crestwood had not quite recently made due; it had flourished despite affliction.

The newly discovered soul of Crestwood didn't be ignored. The account of the town's resurrection spread all over, catching the consideration of news sources, scientists, and adjoining networks. Crestwood turned into an image of trust, a reference point for those confronting comparable difficulties. The town's process was recorded in articles, narratives, and, surprisingly, scholarly examinations, rousing others to have faith in the groundbreaking force of strength.

As the years passed, Crestwood kept on advancing. The scars of the fire blurred out of spotlight, supplanted by a scene that bore the engravings of both the past and the present. The wall painting on the Zenith Assembling Plant stayed a demonstration of the town's excursion, a living heritage that recounted an account of misfortune, diligence, and win.

Crestwood's experience filled in as an update that misfortune, however difficult, could be an impetus for development. The town had confronted the blazes and arisen more grounded, more joined than any time in recent memory. The illustrations learned in the pot of the fire turned into the establishment for a local area that wouldn't be characterized by its scars.

Eventually, Crestwood's story was not just about defeating a solitary catastrophe; it was tied in with embracing change, encouraging versatility, and building a future that mirrored the aggregate soul of its kin. The town had come to life, not as a simple survivor but rather as a living demonstration of the exceptional limit of people to meet up and make something wonderful out of the remains.

### 1.1 Introduction to the pervasive nature of smoking in society

Smoking, with its rings profoundly entwined in the structure holding the system together, remains as an unavoidable and complex peculiarity that has woven itself into the actual embodiment of human life. From social ceremonies to individual propensities, the demonstration of smoking has risen above simple utilization to turn into a diverse articulation, at the same time intelligent of social standards, individual decisions, and cultural designs.

The appeal of smoking stretches out past the limits of individual choices, venturing into the domains of history, brain science, and general wellbeing, making a permanent imprint on the shared perspective.

The foundations of smoking stretch back through the records of time, stringing themselves into the woven artwork of different societies and developments. Whether in the stylized lines of Local American clans, the opium caves of old China, or the tobacco fields of the American South, the demonstration of smoking has appeared in bunch structures, frequently expecting jobs of ceremonial importance or restorative utility. Over hundreds of years, the social and representative elements of smoking developed, entwining with strict practices, social collaborations, and soul changing experiences.

In the cutting edge time, smoking has risen above its verifiable and social settings to turn into a worldwide peculiarity, a propensity that knows no limits of geology, financial status, or age. The pervasive presence of cigarettes and other tobacco items authenticates their standardization inside society. Smoking isn't simply a lone demonstration; it is a common encounter, partook in get-togethers, working environments, and public spaces. The crest of smoke floating through the air act as quiet couriers of a propensity that has become imbued in the regular routines of people all over the planet.

The purposes for the unavoidable idea of smoking are just about as different as the people who participate in this custom. For some's purposes, smoking is a demonstration of resistance, an emblematic motion that challenges cultural standards and assumptions. The cigarette, with its relationship of resistance and rebelliousness, turns into a device of self-articulation, a method for cutting out a personality in a world that frequently requests similarity. For other people, smoking is a survival technique, a shelter in snapshots of stress, uneasiness, or distress. The demonstration of lighting a cigarette turns into a custom of comfort, giving a concise reprieve from the tensions of life.

Besides, the showcasing techniques utilized by tobacco organizations play had a vital impact in propagating the predominance of smoking. Promotions have handily woven pictures of charm, refinement, and disobedience around the demonstration of smoking, making an enchanting charm that rises above the physical and wellbeing related results. The actual bundling turns into a material for sly plan, quietly passing on messages of joy and fulfillment. The purposeful relationship of smoking with beneficial qualities has added to its standardization, making it a propensity as well as an optimistic direction for living for some.

The mental parts of smoking further highlight its inescapable nature. Nicotine, the drug tracked down in tobacco, follows up on the mind's prize framework, making a pattern of reliance that rises above objective navigation. The delight got from smoking becomes interwoven with day to day schedules, making it a troublesome propensity to break.

The customs related with smoking — the flick of a lighter, the material experience of holding a cigarette — add layers of intricacy to the mental connection, changing it into in excess of a basic propensity yet a ceremonial conduct profoundly implanted in the psyche.

The inescapable idea of smoking stretches out past the person to include more extensive cultural designs and approaches. Regardless of the factual wellbeing gambles related with smoking, tobacco stays a legitimate and open item in many regions of the planet. The monetary interests attached to the tobacco business, combined with the income created through charges on tobacco items, make a complicated snare of motivating forces that add to the proceeded with legitimateness and accessibility of cigarettes. The exchange between financial contemplations, political impact, and general wellbeing concerns shapes the scene inside which smoking perseveres.

Normal practices and social mentalities further add to the entrenchment of smoking in the public arena. In certain societies, smoking is profoundly imbued in customary practices and soul changing experiences, making a feeling of coherence and having a place. The public demonstration of smoking fills in as a social paste, cultivating associations and supporting gathering characters. Endeavors to challenge these imbued standards frequently face obstruction, as smoking becomes a singular decision as well as an aggregate demeanor of personality and shared encounters.

Additionally, the depiction of smoking in mainstream society adds one more layer to its unavoidable presence. Films, network shows, and promotions frequently portray smoking as a signifier of insubordination, complexity, or charm. The relationship of smoking with famous figures and characters further implants it in the aggregate creative mind, making a story where smoking isn't simply a propensity however an image of specific prime examples and ways of life. The force of visual narrating reaches out past simple portrayal; it shapes insights and impacts perspectives, adding to the propagation of smoking as a normal practice.

The wellbeing ramifications of smoking, notwithstanding, cast a long shadow over its unavoidable presence. The connection among smoking and a bunch of ailments, including cellular breakdown in the lungs, coronary illness, and respiratory problems, is deep rooted. The cost for general wellbeing is faltering, with smoking-related sicknesses forcing a significant weight on medical care frameworks all over the planet. Regardless of the far reaching dispersal of data about the wellbeing gambles, smoking keeps on being a main source of preventable demise universally.

Endeavors to control smoking and relieve its effect on general wellbeing have taken different structures, going from public mindfulness missions to official measures. Cautioning names on cigarette bundling, against smoking commercials, and smoking suspension programs expect to illuminate and prevent people from taking part in this propensity. However, the profoundly dug in nature of smoking in the public eye represents a considerable test to these drives.

The habit-forming nature of nicotine, combined with the social and mental components of smoking, renders it impervious to regular techniques for intercession.

Smoking discontinuance, in this way, requires a complex methodology that tends to the singular's reliance on nicotine as well as the more extensive social, social, and financial variables that add to the steadiness of smoking. Extensive tobacco control arrangements, including measures like expanded tax assessment, publicizing limitations, and without smoke conditions, expect to establish a climate that beats smoking at both the individual and cultural levels down. Be that as it may, the viability of such arrangements relies on their execution and implementation, which frequently face resistance from strong tobacco entryways and social inactivity.

General wellbeing efforts assume a critical part in testing the standardization of smoking and changing cultural discernments. By dispersing data about the wellbeing dangers of smoking and exposing legends related with the propensity, these missions look to make a change in open cognizance. The objective isn't only to deter current smokers however to keep new ages from surrendering to the charm of smoking. Training turns into an incredible asset in destroying the romanticized pictures encompassing smoking and supplanting them with an unmistakable rude awakening about the wellbeing results.

Local area based mediations likewise assume an essential part in tending to the unavoidable idea of smoking. Support gatherings, guiding administrations, and smoking discontinuance programs offer people a pathway out of fixation, giving the devices and assets expected to break liberated from the pattern of reliance. These mediations perceive the unpredictable transaction between the individual, their social climate, and the more extensive social setting. By encouraging a feeling of local area and understanding, they expect to unravel the snare of variables that add to the propagation of smoking.

The worldwide scene of smoking, in any case, stays dynamic and impervious to simple arrangements. While certain locales have taken huge steps in diminishing smoking rates through extensive tobacco control measures, others wrestle with increasing rates driven by variables like populace development, remiss guidelines, and forceful advertising by the tobacco business. Overcoming any barrier among mindfulness and activity requires a purposeful exertion on various fronts, enveloping public strategy, medical care framework, and cultural perspectives.

All in all, the unavoidable idea of smoking in the public eye mirrors a complicated transaction of verifiable, social, mental, and monetary variables. From its foundations in old customs to its cutting edge manifestation as a worldwide peculiarity, smoking has developed into a complex articulation that rises above individual decisions to shape cultural standards.

The difficulties presented by smoking stretch out past wellbeing contemplations, venturing into the domains of financial matters, legislative issues, and social personality.

Tending to the unavoidable idea of smoking requires an exhaustive and nuanced approach that perceives the interconnectedness of individual way of behaving and more extensive cultural designs. General wellbeing drives, authoritative measures, and local area based mediations should work pair to destroy the settled in designs that add to the determination of smoking. As society wrestles with the results of this unavoidable propensity, the excursion toward a sans smoke future requests aggregate exertion, informed navigation, and an immovable obligation to reshaping the story around smoking.

**1.2 Statistics on global tobacco consumption**

The measurements encompassing worldwide tobacco utilization paint a distinct and sobering image of a propensity profoundly settled in the existences of millions. In spite of boundless consciousness of the wellbeing chances related with smoking, tobacco use stays a common worldwide peculiarity, influencing people across different socioeconomics and geologies. These measurements not just revealed insight into the sheer size of tobacco utilization yet in addition highlight the earnest requirement for extensive endeavors to address the complex difficulties presented by this unavoidable propensity.

As of the latest information accessible, it is assessed that over 1.1 billion individuals overall are standard smokers. This stunning figure addresses a huge piece of the worldwide populace, featuring the broad idea of tobacco use. The ramifications of such inescapable utilization reach out past individual wellbeing worries to incorporate more extensive cultural, financial, and general wellbeing challenges.

Geologically, the circulation of tobacco utilization is lopsided, with specific areas encountering higher commonness rates than others. In some major league salary nations, coordinated endeavors to check smoking have brought about a decrease in commonness rates. In any case, this positive pattern is balanced by increasing paces of tobacco use in low-and center pay nations, where tobacco control measures might be less rigid, and the tobacco business frequently utilizes forceful showcasing techniques to advance its items.

Asia, specifically, stands apart as a locale with high tobacco utilization rates. Nations like China and India, with their enormous populaces, contribute altogether to the worldwide weight of tobacco use. The social meaning of tobacco in a few Asian social orders, combined with the impact of the tobacco business, has added to the constancy of smoking notwithstanding expanded consciousness of its wellbeing results. Essentially, in specific African countries, tobacco use is on the ascent, introducing a disturbing pattern that requires designated mediation.

The effect of tobacco utilization goes past individual wellbeing to apply a significant monetary cost for social orders. The World Wellbeing Association (WHO) appraises that the worldwide financial expense of smoking surpasses trillions of dollars yearly. This financial weight incorporates not just direct medical services costs connected with treating smoking-related ailments yet in addition backhanded costs, for example, lost efficiency because of disease and unexpected passing. The financial repercussions of tobacco use make a powerful case for extensive tobacco control estimates that work on general wellbeing as well as reduce the burden on medical services frameworks and economies.

Besides, the socioeconomics of tobacco use uncover designs that request consideration. While smoking rates among men have customarily been higher than among ladies, the orientation hole is limiting, especially in more youthful age gatherings. In certain districts, young ladies are progressively taking up smoking, highlighting the requirement for designated avoidance and suspension methodologies that address the particular elements of orientation and smoking.

The ascent of elective tobacco and nicotine items likewise adds to the developing scene of tobacco utilization. Items like electronic cigarettes (e-cigarettes) and warmed tobacco gadgets have acquired ubiquity, particularly among more youthful populaces. While these items are in many cases promoted as less unsafe options in contrast to customary cigarettes, their drawn out wellbeing impacts stay a subject of continuous exploration and discussion. The rise of novel tobacco items adds intricacy to the test of directing and controlling tobacco use actually.

Understanding the pervasiveness of tobacco utilization is just a single part of the bigger story. Similarly significant is perceiving the wellbeing effect of smoking on people and populaces. Tobacco use is a main source of preventable passing universally, adding to a variety of illnesses and conditions. Boss among these is cardiovascular illness, with smoking being a significant gamble factor for respiratory failures and strokes. Furthermore, smoking is the essential driver of persistent obstructive pneumonic sickness (COPD), an ever-evolving lung condition that debilitates breathing and fundamentally decreases personal satisfaction.

Maybe most famously, tobacco use is the main source of cellular breakdown in the lungs. The connection among smoking and cellular breakdown in the lungs is deep rooted, with most of cellular breakdown in the lungs cases owing to tobacco openness. The cost for respiratory wellbeing stretches out past malignant growth to incorporate circumstances like emphysema and persistent bronchitis, aggregately known as constant obstructive pneumonic sickness (COPD).

The effect of smoking isn't restricted to the respiratory and cardiovascular frameworks. It stretches out to different organs and frameworks, expanding the gamble of different tumors, including those of the mouth, throat, throat, pancreas, bladder, and cervix. Also, smoking adds to the advancement of type 2 diabetes, demolishes results for people with asthma, and speeds up the maturing system of the skin, prompting untimely kinks.

One of the gravest parts of tobacco's cost for wellbeing is its effect on maternal and youngster wellbeing. Maternal smoking during pregnancy is related with an elevated gamble of complexities, for example, preterm birth, low birth weight, and unexpected baby passing condition (SIDS). The openness of youngsters to handed-down cigarette smoke, whether in utero or in the home climate, represents a huge wellbeing risk, impeding lung improvement and improving the probability of respiratory contaminations.

The worldwide weight of sickness owing to tobacco is significant. As indicated by the WHO, tobacco use kills in excess of 8 million individuals every year, with in excess of 7 million of those passings being the consequence of direct tobacco use and roughly 1.2 million due to non-smokers being presented to handed-down cigarette smoke. These figures highlight the critical requirement for deliberate endeavors to diminish tobacco utilization and alleviate the overwhelming wellbeing outcomes related with smoking.

Endeavors to battle tobacco utilization have taken different structures, incorporating both public and worldwide drives. The Structure Show on Tobacco Control (FCTC), a worldwide settlement embraced by the World Wellbeing Gathering, addresses a milestone work to address the worldwide tobacco pandemic. The FCTC gives an exhaustive system to tobacco control, including measures connected with cost and expense strategies, security from openness to handed-down cigarette smoke, bundling and naming of tobacco items, and public mindfulness crusades.

Nations that are gatherings to the FCTC have focused on carrying out these proof based measures to decrease tobacco utilization and safeguard general wellbeing. In any case, the adequacy of these actions relies upon the degree to which they are taken on and authorized at the public level. A few nations have taken huge steps in executing tobacco control strategies, bringing about decreases in smoking rates. Be that as it may, others face difficulties in defeating obstruction from the tobacco business and tending to imbued social standards related with smoking.

One of the key methodologies illustrated in the FCTC is the execution of tobacco tax collection arrangements to build the cost of tobacco items. More exorbitant costs have been displayed to dissuade smoking inception, support end, and decrease generally tobacco utilization. Nonetheless, the adequacy of tax collection approaches is dependent upon their plan, with elements, for example, the greatness of assessment builds, the design of tax collection, and the accessibility of reasonable choices affecting their effect.

Past tax assessment, the guideline of tobacco publicizing, advancement, and sponsorship is one more basic part of tobacco control endeavors. The tobacco business has a long history of utilizing modern showcasing methodologies to advance its items, especially to youngsters. Far reaching prohibitions on tobacco promoting, combined with realistic wellbeing admonitions on bundling, plan to balance the business' endeavors to glamorize and standardize smoking.

Sans smoke strategies, which forbid smoking in indoor public spaces, working environments, and certain outside regions, address one more essential device in diminishing openness to handed-down cigarette smoke and establishing conditions that put smoking down. The execution of sans smoke approaches has been related with critical decreases in smoking pervasiveness and enhancements in respiratory wellbeing.

Schooling and mindfulness crusades assume an essential part in changing cultural view of smoking and scattering fantasies encompassing tobacco use. These missions intend to illuminate the general population about the wellbeing dangers of smoking, expose the charm related with tobacco items, and advance discontinuance assets. Designated drives that address explicit populaces, like youngsters, pregnant ladies, and people with low financial status, are fundamental in fitting messages to different crowds.

Smoking end programs, offering backing and assets for people hoping to stop smoking, are a basic part of exhaustive tobacco control endeavors. These projects might incorporate directing administrations, pharmacological mediations, and local area based drives. Quitlines, online assets, and versatile applications give open roads to people looking for help with their excursion toward tobacco discontinuance.

Notwithstanding these multi-layered endeavors, challenges continue accomplishing significant decreases in tobacco utilization worldwide. The tobacco business' proceeded with impact, especially in low-and center pay nations, represents an impressive deterrent to powerful tobacco control. Forceful showcasing strategies, item advancement, and lawful difficulties to tobacco control measures are among the techniques utilized by the business to keep up with and extend its portion of the overall industry.

**1.3 Overview of the health risks associated with smoking**

The wellbeing chances related with smoking structure a complete and disturbing scene, uncovering the complex cost that tobacco use claims on the human body. Smoking is evidently connected to a bunch of inconvenient wellbeing results, influencing essentially every organ framework and contributing fundamentally to a scope of dangerous circumstances. From respiratory infirmities to cardiovascular sicknesses and different tumors, the outcomes of smoking saturate the whole of a singular's prosperity and reach out to more extensive general wellbeing concerns.

Cellular breakdown in the lungs remains as one of the most deep rooted and famous wellbeing chances related with smoking. The connection between tobacco use and cellular breakdown in the lungs is unequivocal, with most of cellular breakdown in the lungs cases owing to smoking. The cancer-causing agents present in tobacco smoke, including polycyclic sweet-smelling hydrocarbons and nitrosamines, penetrate the sensitive tissues of the lungs, starting a fountain of hereditary changes that can come full circle in the uncontrolled development of threatening cells.

The slippery idea of cellular breakdown in the lungs lies in its not unexpected asymptomatic beginning phases, prompting deferred finding and less fortunate forecasts. As the infection advances, side effects, for example, relentless hack, chest agony, and windedness might show. When these side effects become clear, the malignant growth might have progressed to a phase where corrective intercessions are less viable. Cellular breakdown in the lungs addresses an imposing test in the domain of general wellbeing, with a high death rate and huge medical care troubles.

Past cellular breakdown in the lungs, smoking causes a significant effect for respiratory wellbeing, adding to a range of conditions that compromise the usefulness of the respiratory framework. Constant obstructive pneumonic sickness (COPD), an aggregate term including persistent bronchitis and emphysema, is a great representation. COPD is portrayed by moderate wind current limit and irreversible harm to lung tissue, bringing about side effects like ongoing hack, extreme bodily fluid creation, and shortness of breath.

The pathophysiology of COPD is unpredictably connected to the inward breath of destructive substances present in tobacco smoke. The ongoing aggravation prompted by these substances prompts primary changes in the aviation routes and alveoli, blocking the progression of air and compromising the trading of oxygen and carbon dioxide. People with COPD experience a steady disintegration in lung capability, affecting their capacity to take part in routine exercises and lessening their personal satisfaction.

Smoking isn't just an essential gamble factor for COPD yet additionally fuels the movement of the infection. Proceeded with tobacco use among people with COPD worsens irritation, speeds up the decrease in lung capability, and builds the recurrence and seriousness of intensifications. COPD addresses a significant weight on medical care frameworks, with critical financial expenses credited to hospitalizations, drugs, and related medical care use.

Notwithstanding lung-related conditions, smoking demands a weighty cost for cardiovascular wellbeing, adding to a scope of sicknesses that all in all comprise a main source of bleakness and mortality worldwide. Atherosclerosis, the gradual limiting and solidifying of conduits, is a trademark result of smoking on cardiovascular wellbeing. The synthetic substances in tobacco smoke advance the arrangement of blood vessel plaques, comprising of cholesterol, greasy stores, and fiery cells.

Atherosclerosis makes way for a bunch of cardiovascular intricacies, including coronary corridor illness (computer aided design), myocardial localized necrosis (respiratory failure), and fringe blood vessel infection (Cushion). Computer aided design happens when the coronary conduits, which supply blood to the heart muscle, become restricted or hindered, prompting ischemia and possibly deadly results. Myocardial localized necrosis happens when a coronary supply route is totally hindered, bringing about the passing of a piece of the heart muscle.

Fringe blood vessel sickness, described by diminished blood stream to the appendages, can prompt claudication (torment with strolling), non-mending wounds, and, in serious cases, appendage removals. The harmful impacts of smoking on the cardiovascular framework are not restricted to the conduits; they stretch out to the heart's beat and capability. Smoking expands the gamble of arrhythmias, like atrial fibrillation, and adds to cardiovascular breakdown, a condition where the heart's capacity to siphon blood is compromised.

Besides, smoking significantly affects pulse, further intensifying the gamble of cardiovascular occasions. Nicotine, a critical part of tobacco, invigorates the arrival of adrenaline and other pressure chemicals, prompting an expansion in pulse and circulatory strain. Constant openness to these cardiovascular stressors adds to the improvement of hypertension, a critical gamble factor for coronary illness and stroke.

The interlacing connection among smoking and cardiovascular wellbeing highlights the gravity of tobacco's effect on generally prosperity. Cardiovascular sicknesses, all in all liable for a significant piece of worldwide passings, comprise a significant general wellbeing challenge. Tending to the wellbeing gambles related with smoking requires a far reaching approach that includes both tobacco control measures and techniques to relieve the cardiovascular results of smoking.

The impeding impacts of smoking reach out to different organs and frameworks, leading to a different cluster of malignant growths that burden people who participate in tobacco use. The cancer-causing nature of tobacco smoke opens the body to a mixed drink of hurtful substances that start hereditary transformations and cell changes helpful for the improvement of malignancies. Among the diseases connected to smoking are those influencing the mouth, throat, throat, pancreas, bladder, cervix, and kidneys.

The components through which smoking adds to these different tumors are multilayered. On account of cellular breakdown in the lungs, the inward breath of cancer-causing agents straightforwardly opens lung tissue to unsafe substances, starting the change of sound cells into harmful ones. For malignant growths of the stomach related and urinary parcels, the immediate contact of tobacco smoke with these tissues during smoking and ingestion of tobacco items adds to the cancer-causing process.

Cigarette smoking is a perceived reason for pancreatic disease, an especially forceful threat with a high death rate. The relationship among smoking and pancreatic malignant growth is deeply grounded, with studies demonstrating that drawn out smokers face a fundamentally raised hazard of fostering this destructive infection. The exact instruments through which smoking adds to pancreatic disease are complicated and may include both immediate and aberrant pathways.

Likewise, smoking is a critical gamble factor for bladder disease, with the cancer-causing agents in tobacco smoke entering the circulation system and in the long run being sifted by the kidneys. The discharge of these cancer-causing agents in pee uncovered the bladder coating to unsafe substances, adding to the improvement of dangerous sores. The elevated gamble of bladder malignant growth among smokers highlights the unavoidable effect of tobacco use on different organs and frameworks inside the body.

Smoking's harmful consequences for regenerative wellbeing reach out past the person to influence maternal and fetal prosperity. Maternal smoking during pregnancy is related with a reiteration of unfriendly results, all things considered known as maternal smoking condition. These results incorporate an expanded gamble of preterm birth, low birth weight, stillbirth, and unexpected baby passing condition (SIDS).

The unsafe outcomes of maternal smoking are credited to the entry of harmful substances from the mother's circulation system to the creating embryo through the placenta. Nicotine, carbon monoxide, and other hurtful synthetic compounds present in tobacco smoke can debilitate fetal development, prevent organ advancement, and compromise the oxygen supply to the creating embryo. The repercussions of maternal smoking resonate through the existence course of the kid, affecting respiratory wellbeing, mental capability, and vulnerability to different ailments.

Notwithstanding its effect on pregnancy results, smoking represents a critical danger to richness and conceptive wellbeing. Both male and female smokers experience disturbances in conceptive capability that can hinder their capacity to consider. In men, smoking is related with diminished sperm quality, changed sperm motility, and an expanded gamble of erectile brokenness. In ladies, smoking can disturb the hormonal equilibrium, impede ovulation, and add to conditions like barrenness and early menopause.

The impacts of smoking on regenerative wellbeing reach out to the post pregnancy time frame, influencing breastfeeding results. Maternal smoking has been related with a decrease in bosom milk creation and changes in the sythesis of bosom milk. The presence of nicotine and other destructive substances in bosom milk can open babies to extra wellbeing gambles, underlining the significance of smoking discontinuance during pregnancy and breastfeeding.

The wellbeing gambles related with smoking are not exclusively restricted to the actual domain; they likewise reach out to the psychological wellness and prosperity of people who participate in tobacco use. Arising proof proposes a bidirectional connection among smoking and psychological wellness problems, with smoking filling in as both a supporter of and an outcome of emotional well-being difficulties.

The wellbeing gambles related with smoking comprise a mind boggling and complex scene, incorporating a wide exhibit of negative impacts that resonate all through the body. Smoking, essentially connected to the inward breath of tobacco smoke, is a significant general wellbeing worry that contributes fundamentally to dreariness and mortality around the world. From respiratory and cardiovascular difficulties to different malignant growths and regenerative wellbeing challenges, the results of tobacco use stretch out across for all intents and purposes each organ framework, highlighting the earnest requirement for far reaching tobacco control measures and smoking suspension intercessions.

At the very front of the wellbeing gambles related with smoking is the unavoidable connection to respiratory sicknesses, with ongoing obstructive pneumonic infection (COPD) remaining as an unmistakable model. COPD includes ongoing bronchitis and emphysema, the two of which are portrayed by moderate and irreversible harm to the aviation routes and lung tissue. The inward breath of harmful substances present in tobacco smoke, including particulate matter and poisonous gases, starts an outpouring of provocative reactions inside the lungs, prompting primary changes and weakened lung capability.

People with constant bronchitis experience industrious irritation of the aviation routes, joined by side effects like persistent hack, unnecessary creation of bodily fluid, and intermittent respiratory contaminations. The persistent aggravation and irritation add to the restricting of the aviation routes, obstructing the progression of air and hindering the typical freedom of bodily fluid. These progressions reduce respiratory capability as well as increment the weakness to respiratory contaminations, further fueling the weight on impacted people.

Emphysema, one more part of COPD, includes the annihilation of the alveoli — the little air sacs answerable for gas trade in the lungs. The continuous breakdown of alveolar walls diminishes the surface region accessible for oxygen and carbon dioxide trade, debilitating the lungs' capacity to oxygenate the blood satisfactorily. People with emphysema frequently experience shortness of breath, particularly during actual effort, as the compromised lung capability restricts their ability for oxygen take-up.

The synergistic effect of persistent bronchitis and emphysema on respiratory wellbeing is significant, adding to a descending winding of demolishing side effects, diminished practice resilience, and a general decrease in personal satisfaction. COPD is a main source of incapacity and mortality worldwide, putting a significant weight on medical care frameworks and highlighting the basic of smoking suspension as an essential preventive measure.

Inseparably connected to COPD is the increased gamble of respiratory contaminations among smokers. The compromised respiratory guards coming about because of smoking-initiated lung harm establish a climate helpful for diseases. Smokers are more defenseless to respiratory contaminations like pneumonia, bronchitis, and flu, with diseases frequently prompting more serious and delayed ailment contrasted with non-smokers.

Cellular breakdown in the lungs, maybe the most famous wellbeing risk related with smoking, is a significant supporter of disease related passings around the world. The cancer-causing intensifies present in tobacco smoke, including polycyclic fragrant hydrocarbons and nitrosamines, straightforwardly harm the DNA inside lung cells, setting off hereditary transformations that can prompt the uncontrolled development of dangerous cells. Cellular breakdown in the lungs frequently advances treacherously, with side effects appearing in later stages when the sickness is less agreeable to healing mediations.

The connection among smoking and cellular breakdown in the lungs is hearty, with most of cellular breakdown in the lungs cases credited to tobacco use. The gamble of creating cellular breakdown in the lungs is straightforwardly corresponding to the length and force of smoking, underlining the aggregate and portion subordinate nature of tobacco-related carcinogenesis. Past the lungs, smoking is likewise ensnared in tumors influencing different organs, including the mouth, throat, throat, pancreas, bladder, cervix, and kidneys.

Esophageal malignant growth, for example, is firmly connected with smoking, especially when joined with weighty liquor utilization — a cooperative energy that enhances the cancer-causing impacts. The immediate contact of tobacco smoke with the esophageal coating adds to the advancement of precancerous sores and malignancies. Essentially, the relationship among smoking and pancreatic disease highlights the diverse effect of tobacco on various organ frameworks, with pancreatic malignant growth addressing an especially forceful and deadly threat.

The urological outcomes of smoking are clear in the elevated gamble of bladder disease among people who take part in tobacco use. Cancer-causing agents present in tobacco smoke are separated by the kidneys and discharged in pee, uncovering the bladder covering to hurtful substances. The outcome is an expanded weakness to the improvement of dangerous sores inside the bladder, requiring a thorough comprehension of the interconnectedness between tobacco use and different malignant growth types.

Conceptive wellbeing isn't saved from the inescapable wellbeing gambles related with smoking. Maternal smoking during pregnancy represents a critical danger to both maternal and fetal prosperity, adding to a group of stars of unfavorable results all things considered known as maternal smoking condition. Pregnant ladies who smoke face a raised gamble of preterm birth, low birth weight, stillbirth, and abrupt newborn child passing condition (SIDS).

The poisonous substances present in tobacco smoke, including nicotine and carbon monoxide, cross the placenta and enter the fetal circulatory system, applying adverse impacts on fetal turn of events. Nicotine, specifically, tightens veins, diminishing the progression of oxygen and supplements to the creating hatchling. This decreased oxygen supply can hinder fetal development, prompting low birth weight and expanding the gamble of intricacies during and after conveyance.

Additionally, maternal smoking is ensnared in the disturbance of neurodevelopment, with long haul ramifications for the mental and conduct results of the uncovered posterity. Kids brought into the world to moms who smoked during pregnancy might confront an expanded gamble of consideration shortfall/hyperactivity jumble (ADHD), learning incapacities, and conduct issues. The unavoidable effect of maternal smoking stretches out past the quick perinatal period, featuring the requirement for designated mediations to help smoking suspension during pregnancy.

The injurious impacts of smoking on conceptive wellbeing stretch out to post pregnancy periods, influencing breastfeeding results. Maternal smoking is related with a decrease in bosom milk creation and modifications in the organization of bosom milk. The presence of nicotine and other hurtful substances in bosom milk can open babies to extra wellbeing chances, highlighting the significance of smoking end during breastfeeding to streamline the wellbeing and prosperity of the two moms and newborn children.

Cardiovascular infections, on the whole liable for a critical extent of worldwide dismalness and mortality, comprise one more significant class of wellbeing gambles related with smoking. The effect of smoking on cardiovascular wellbeing is diverse, adding to the turn of events and movement of atherosclerosis, coronary vein sickness (computer aided design), myocardial localized necrosis (cardiovascular failure), fringe blood vessel illness (Cushion), arrhythmias, and cardiovascular breakdown.

Atherosclerosis, the sign of cardiovascular illness, includes the progressive limiting and solidifying of veins because of the testimony of cholesterol, greasy stores, and provocative cells. Smoking speeds up the movement of atherosclerosis through various components, including the advancement of endothelial brokenness, aggravation, and oxidative pressure. The combined impact is the development of blood vessel plaques that obstruct blood stream, compromise oxygen conveyance to fundamental organs, and make a prolific ground for cardiovascular occasions.

Coronary corridor illness, a typical indication of atherosclerosis influencing the veins providing blood to the heart, is complicatedly connected to smoking. The openness to destructive synthetics in tobacco smoke adds to the development of coronary plaques, prompting the restricting of coronary corridors and a diminished limit with regards to blood stream. This compromised blood stream makes way for angina (chest torment) and, in serious cases, myocardial localized necrosis (coronary episode), wherein the blood supply to a piece of the heart muscle is suddenly cut off, bringing about tissue harm and potential cardiovascular breakdown.

Fringe blood vessel infection, portrayed by diminished blood stream to the appendages, is one more outcome of smoking-incited atherosclerosis. People with fringe blood vessel sickness might encounter claudication (torment with strolling), non-recuperating wounds, and an expanded gamble of removals.

The effect of smoking on the fringe supply routes mirrors the foundational idea of atherosclerosis, highlighting the requirement for thorough cardiovascular gamble decrease systems in people who smoke.

Smoking applies significant consequences for the mood and capability of the heart, adding to arrhythmias and cardiovascular breakdown. Nicotine, a critical part of tobacco, animates the arrival of adrenaline and other pressure chemicals, prompting an expansion in pulse and circulatory strain. Constant openness to these cardiovascular stressors disturbs the ordinary electrical movement of the heart, inclining people toward arrhythmias like atrial fibrillation.

Moreover, smoking-initiated oxidative pressure and irritation add to the improvement of cardiovascular breakdown — a condition where the heart's capacity to siphon blood is compromised. The unfriendly effect of smoking on the cardiovascular framework isn't restricted to the actual heart; it stretches out to veins, expanding the gamble of apoplexy (blood cluster arrangement) and worsening the atherosclerotic interaction.

Notwithstanding the prompt and direct wellbeing chances related with smoking, the propensity likewise applies a significant effect on psychological wellness and prosperity. Arising proof recommends a bidirectional connection among smoking and psychological wellness issues, with smoking filling in as both a supporter of and an outcome of emotional well-being difficulties.

People with psychological wellness conditions, like misery, nervousness, and substance use issues, are lopsidedly bound to smoke than those without such circumstances. Smoking frequently turns into a maladaptive survival strategy for people wrestling with mental trouble, stress, and inner commotion. The psychoactive impacts of nicotine, which can briefly reduce side effects of nervousness and sorrow, further add to the foundation of smoking as a survival method.

On the other hand, smoking has been recognized as a gamble factor for the turn of events and worsening of emotional well-being problems. The neurobiological impacts of nicotine on synapse frameworks, especially dopamine, serotonin, and norepinephrine, may impact temperament guideline and add to the weakness to psychological wellness challenges. Longitudinal investigations have exhibited an expanded gamble of creating state of mind and uneasiness problems among people who smoke, highlighting the perplexing transaction among smoking and psychological well-being.

The co-event of smoking and psychological well-being difficulties presents exceptional difficulties for intercession and end endeavors. People with emotional well-being issues might confront obstructions to stopping smoking, remembering an elevated reliance for nicotine, worries about compounding mental side effects, and restricted admittance to smoking end assets.

Tending to the convergence of smoking and emotional well-being requires coordinated approaches that perceive the bidirectional relationship and designer intercessions to the particular necessities of people with emotional wellness conditions.

The many-sided snare of wellbeing gambles related with smoking highlights the direness of carrying out complete tobacco control measures and smoking suspension intercessions. While the prompt and direct results of smoking on respiratory, cardiovascular, malignant growth related, and conceptive wellbeing are significant, the more extensive cultural effect reaches out to expanded medical services usage, financial weights, and wellbeing differences.

Endeavors to alleviate the wellbeing dangers of smoking have taken different structures, going from general wellbeing efforts and administrative measures to smoking discontinuance projects and global arrangements. The System Show on Tobacco Control (FCTC), embraced by the World Wellbeing Gathering, addresses a milestone worldwide work to battle the worldwide tobacco pestilence. The FCTC gives an exhaustive system to tobacco control, incorporating measures connected with cost and duty strategies, insurance from openness to handed-down cigarette smoke, bundling and marking of tobacco items, and public mindfulness crusades.

Public and territorial tobacco control strategies assume a crucial part in decreasing the pervasiveness of smoking and limiting the related wellbeing gambles. Tobacco tax collection arrangements, which increment the cost of tobacco items, have been demonstrated to be powerful in diminishing smoking commencement, advancing suspension, and controlling generally speaking tobacco utilization. Nonetheless, the effect of tax collection strategies relies upon their size, structure, and the accessibility of reasonable other options.

Guideline of tobacco publicizing, advancement, and sponsorship is one more basic part of tobacco control endeavors. The tobacco business has a past filled with utilizing modern showcasing methodologies to glamorize and standardize smoking, especially among youngsters. Extensive restrictions on tobacco promoting, combined with realistic wellbeing alerts on bundling, mean to balance the business' endeavors and decrease the charm of tobacco items.

Without smoke strategies, disallowing smoking in indoor public spaces, working environments, and certain open air regions, address a critical device in diminishing openness to handed-down cigarette smoke and establishing conditions that put smoking down. The execution of sans smoke strategies has been related with huge decreases in smoking pervasiveness and upgrades in respiratory wellbeing.

Training and mindfulness crusades comprise a fundamental component of tobacco control systems, intending to illuminate general society about the wellbeing dangers of smoking, scatter fantasies encompassing tobacco use, and advance smoking suspension assets.

Designated drives that address explicit populaces, like youngsters, pregnant ladies, and people with low financial status, are instrumental in fitting messages to different crowds and diminishing wellbeing differences.

Smoking end programs, offering backing and assets for people hoping to stop smoking, are basic in tending to the fixation and reliance related with tobacco use. These projects might incorporate directing administrations, pharmacological mediations, and local area based drives. Quitlines, online assets, and versatile applications give available roads to people looking for help with their excursion toward tobacco suspension.

Regardless of these complex endeavors, challenges continue accomplishing significant decreases in tobacco utilization around the world. The tobacco business' proceeded with impact, especially in low-and center pay nations, represents an imposing hindrance to successful tobacco control. Forceful advertising strategies, item advancement, and legitimate difficulties to tobacco control measures are among the procedures utilized by the business to keep up with and grow its piece of the pie.

Additionally, the scene of tobacco utilization is developing with the ascent of new and arising tobacco and nicotine items. Electronic cigarettes (e-cigarettes) and warmed tobacco gadgets, frequently advertised as less destructive options in contrast to customary cigarettes, have acquired fame, particularly among more youthful populaces. The security and long haul wellbeing impacts of these original items remain subjects of progressing examination and discussion, featuring the powerful idea of the tobacco scene and the requirement for versatile administrative systems.

# Chapter 2

### Origins and Influence

The starting points and impact of any social, cultural, or verifiable peculiarity are many times unpredictable and diverse, formed by a bunch of interconnected factors that wind around together to make a mind boggling embroidery. Such is the situation with the starting points and impact of different components that have made a permanent imprint on the human experience. These components, whether they be social practices, philosophies, or mechanical advancements, are in many cases profoundly implanted in the shared perspective of social orders, affecting convictions, ways of behaving, and the direction of human turn of events.

One remarkable illustration of a social practice with significant beginnings and impact is the specialty of narrating. From old oral customs to present day writing and computerized media, narrating has been a basic part of human correspondence and culture. The underlying foundations of narrating can be followed back to ancient times when early people, without composed language, depended on oral accounts to share information, communicate social qualities, and figure out their general surroundings.

In the beginning phases of human progress, narrating filled in as an essential method for protecting history, passing down shrewdness, and encouraging a feeling of shared character. Fantasies, legends, and incredible stories conveyed moral examples, made sense of normal peculiarities, and gave a system to figuring out the intricacies of life. As social orders advanced and created composed dialects, narrating extended its arrive at through composed writing, turning into an incredible asset for molding social stories and impacting cultural standards.

Strict texts, like the Holy book, the Quran, and the Vedas, stand as fantastic instances of the impact of narrating on forming conviction frameworks and social personalities. These texts act as sacrosanct sacred texts as well as archives of moral lessons, core values, and essential stories that have molded the moral structures of whole developments. The effect of strict narrating reaches out past individual beliefs to impact craftsmanship, writing, and, surprisingly, political philosophies.

The Renaissance time frame in Europe denoted a huge defining moment in the development of narrating and social impact. The restoration of traditional learning, the appearance of the print machine, and the democratization of information assumed vital parts in changing the social scene. Crafted by artistic goliaths like William Shakespeare and Miguel de Cervantes engaged crowds as well as tested cultural standards, addressed power, and investigated the profundities of the human experience.

As the world entered the advanced time, the impact of narrating extended dramatically with the coming of broad communications. The improvement of innovations like the print machine, radio, TV, and the web democratized admittance to data and accounts, permitting stories to contact more extensive crowds with exceptional speed and scale. This democratization of narrating had significant ramifications for social trade, social developments, and the molding of shared mindset.

In the domain of political impact, discourses and manner of speaking have been amazing assets over the entire course of time. Pioneers and speakers have utilized the specialty of influence to assemble populaces, articulate dreams, and shape the course of countries. The discourses of figures like Martin Luther Ruler Jr., Winston Churchill, and Nelson Mandela affected the results of verifiable occasions as well as passed on getting through heritages that proceed to motivate and reverberate across ages.

One more powerful power with profound authentic roots is theory. The thoughts and lessons of logicians like Plato, Aristotle, Confucius, and Immanuel Kant have molded the scholarly underpinnings of social orders and affected the advancement of political, moral, and logical idea. The persevering through effect of philosophical request is obvious in the rules that support overall sets of laws, administration structures, and moral systems all over the planet.

Logical revelations and mechanical advancements address one more domain of human undertaking with extensive beginnings and impact. The logical upheaval of the seventeenth hundred years, set apart by figures like Galileo Galilei and Sir Isaac Newton, changed the manner in which humankind grasps the normal world. The resulting progressions in science and innovation, from the Modern Unrest to the Data Age, have reshaped social orders, economies, and day to day existence on a worldwide scale.

The impact of innovation is especially articulated in the contemporary time, where fast progressions in correspondence, transportation, and data have introduced a period of exceptional availability. The web, specifically, has changed how data is scattered, giving a stage to different voices and points of view. Web-based entertainment, a result of the computerized age, has intensified the impact of people and networks, reshaping public talk and testing customary wellsprings of power.

Social peculiarities like music, style, and craftsmanship additionally bear the engraving of their beginnings and apply huge effect on social orders. The advancement of music, from old songs to contemporary kinds, reflects evolving tastes, cultural qualities, and mechanical developments. Likewise, the universe of design fills in as a visual narrative of social movements, reflecting cultural mentalities, characters, and desires.

Workmanship, in its different structures, has been a vehicle for communicating the human experience, testing shows, and starting social developments.

Language itself, as a basic instrument of correspondence and articulation, conveys huge impact. The advancement of dialects, tongues, and semantic articulations is entwined with the social chronicles of networks. Language impacts thought, impacts character, and fills in as a course for protecting and sending social legacy.

The culinary world gives one more focal point through which to investigate beginnings and impact. The relocation of fixings, recipes, and culinary procedures has added to the rich embroidered artwork of worldwide foods. Food, past its job as food, fills in as a social relic, a marker of personality, and a medium through which networks express their extraordinary narratives and customs.

Logical headways in hereditary qualities and antiquarianism have given bits of knowledge into the beginnings and relocations of human populaces, revealing the profound interconnections that connect different societies and developments. The investigation of human DNA has uncovered shared parentage, movement designs, and the mixing of hereditary material over centuries, testing shortsighted stories of social disengagement and featuring the interconnected idea of mankind's set of experiences.

While investigating the beginnings and impact of different social, cultural, and verifiable components, it becomes obvious that these powers are entwined, molding and being formed by each other in a dynamic and equal relationship. The impacts are not bound to discrete classes yet rather cross-over and converge, making a rich and complex mosaic of human experience.

All in all, the starting points and impact of social, cultural, and authentic components are huge and interconnected, mirroring the complex embroidery of the human experience. Whether in the domains of narrating, reasoning, innovation, or cooking, the strings of impact wind through existence, molding convictions, ways of behaving, and the development of social orders. Understanding these starting points gives bits of knowledge into the powers that have molded our reality and the continuous exchange that keeps on impacting the course of mankind's set of experiences.

## 2.1 Historical background of tobacco use

The verifiable foundation of tobacco use is an excursion that traverses hundreds of years and mainlands, set apart by social, monetary, and social moves that have molded the direction of this omnipresent propensity. The starting points of tobacco use are well established in the practices of native people groups, and its ensuing spread across the globe has been entwined with colonization, exchange, and the development of worldwide business sectors.

Tobacco, a plant local to the Americas, holds a sacrosanct spot in the ceremonies and customs of different native societies. Archeological proof proposes that tobacco has been developed and involved by native people groups in the Americas for millennia. The tobacco plant, deductively known as Nicotiana tabacum and Nicotiana rustica, assumed a focal part in strict services, recuperating practices, and get-togethers.

Native people group viewed tobacco as a holy plant with otherworldly importance.

The utilization of tobacco was frequently joined by customs and functions, representing an association with the heavenly, cultivating social securities, and filling in as a course for correspondence with the profound domain. The development and utilization of tobacco were profoundly implanted in the texture of native life, mirroring an agreeable connection among people and nature.

European investigation and the Columbian Trade in the fifteenth and sixteenth hundreds of years assumed a vital part in the worldwide dispersal of tobacco. As European voyagers experienced native societies in the Americas, they noticed and took on the utilization of tobacco in different structures, including smoking, biting, and snuffing. The travelers, including Christopher Columbus and Hernán Cortés, acquainted tobacco with Europe, where it immediately acquired prevalence.

The spread of tobacco in Europe was worked with by different variables, incorporating its relationship with restorative properties and its outlandish charm.

At first utilized for its apparent helpful advantages, tobacco was embraced by European doctors who recommended it for a scope of diseases. The prevalence of smoking tobacco, in any case, rose above its restorative use, and it turned into a popular diversion among the European tip top.

By the seventeenth 100 years, tobacco had solidly set up a good foundation for itself in European social orders, with committed spaces known as tobacco houses or cafés arising as scenes for mingling and getting a charge out of tobacco. The propensity for smoking spread to different social classes, turning into an image of complexity and economic wellbeing. The worldwide exchange tobacco extended quickly, determined by European interest for the yield.

Colonization assumed a critical part in the multiplication of tobacco development and exchange. European powers, especially Spain and Portugal, laid out tobacco estates in their provinces, utilizing the work of oppressed people to develop and handle the harvest. The development of tobacco turned into a foundation of the estate economy in locales like the Caribbean and the American South.

The work serious nature of tobacco development filled the transoceanic slave exchange, as subjugated people from Africa were effectively brought to the Americas to chip away at tobacco ranches. The ruthless double-dealing of subjugated workers added to the monetary outcome of tobacco development yet in addition highlighted the human expense of the tobacco business' extension.

The eighteenth century saw the industrialization of tobacco creation, with developments, for example, the mechanized cigarette-production machine changing the scale and effectiveness of tobacco fabricating. Cigarettes, recently moved manually, turned out to be more open and reasonable, adding to a flood in tobacco utilization. The boundless accessibility of cigarettes established the groundwork for the tobacco business' climb to financial noticeable quality.

As the tobacco business prospered, so did worries about the wellbeing impacts of tobacco use. In the twentieth hundred years, logical examination started to reveal the connections among smoking and different medical issue, including cellular breakdown in the lungs, coronary illness, and respiratory sicknesses. The Top health spokesperson's Report in the US in 1964 assumed a vital part in bringing issues to light about the wellbeing dangers of smoking, denoting a defining moment in open view of tobacco use.

Regardless of the mounting proof of the damages related with tobacco use, the tobacco business utilized refined showcasing methodologies to advance its items. Promoting efforts, supports by superstars, and the presentation of separated cigarettes were among the business' strategies to keep up with and extend its piece of the pie. The depiction of smoking as impressive and socially advantageous persevered, even as general wellbeing efforts tried to counter these stories.

The last 50% of the twentieth century saw a flood in endeavors to direct and control tobacco use. State run administrations all over the planet carried out measures, for example, tobacco charges, smoking boycotts out in the open spaces, and realistic admonition names on cigarette bundling. Worldwide drives, remembering the Structure Show for Tobacco Control (FCTC), looked to arrange worldwide endeavors to check the tobacco scourge.

While these actions have added to decreases in smoking rates in certain districts, the tobacco business keeps on adjusting to evolving conditions. The rise of elective nicotine items, like electronic cigarettes (e-cigarettes), has acquainted new intricacies with the scene of tobacco use. E-cigarettes, promoted as less destructive other options, have acquired prominence, particularly among youngsters.

The worldwide idea of the tobacco business presents difficulties for facilitated guideline and control. In low-and center pay nations, where the tobacco business has extended its range, administrative endeavors are much of the time hampered by monetary contemplations and the impact of strong tobacco organizations. The promoting of tobacco items, especially to youth, stays an unavoidable issue that requires continuous carefulness and intercession.

All in all, the verifiable foundation of tobacco use mirrors a mind boggling exchange of social practices, monetary interests, and worldwide exchange. From its sacrosanct starting points in native societies to its commercialization and industrialization, tobacco has made a permanent imprint on social orders all over the planet. The development of tobacco use has been set apart by both social importance and general wellbeing challenges, with progressing endeavors to address the mind boggling snare of elements that add to its steadiness. Understanding the verifiable setting of tobacco use is fundamental for conceiving extensive methodologies to relieve its effect and diagram a course toward a without tobacco future.

## 2.2 Exploration of cultural and societal influences on smoking

The investigation of social and cultural impacts on smoking uncovers a powerful interchange between individual way of behaving, social standards, and more extensive social designs. Smoking, a training profoundly imbued in numerous social orders across the globe, isn't only an individual decision yet is unpredictably woven into the texture of social customs, social ceremonies, and verifiable settings. Understanding these impacts is critical for creating successful tobacco control procedures that address the complex idea of smoking way of behaving.

Social impacts on smoking manifest in different structures, going from conventional ceremonies to the depiction of smoking in writing, workmanship, and media. In many societies, smoking is entwined with transitional experiences, strict functions, and public get-togethers. The representative meaning of smoking in these settings goes past the simple utilization of tobacco; it turns into a ritualized act that connotes character, social bonds, or profound associations.

For instance, certain native societies consolidate smoking in stylized rehearses for the purpose of correspondence with the otherworldly domain. The demonstration of smoking is saturated with imagery, addressing an association with progenitors, the regular world, or heavenly elements. In such settings, smoking isn't seen exclusively as an individual decision yet as a mutual or holy demonstration that rises above individual way of behaving.

Also, in a few Eastern societies, smoking holds profound social importance. Rehearses like the Japanese tea function might include the sharing of cigarettes as a token of neighborliness and fellowship. The social elements of smoking in these settings add to the standardization and social acknowledgment of the way of behaving, supporting its social roots.

The depiction of smoking in writing, workmanship, and media further enhances its social impact. In writing, smoking has been portrayed as an image of disobedience, refinement, or existential thought. Characters in books and movies what smoke's identity is frequently connected with specific character qualities or cultural mentalities, molding impression of smoking as a statement of independence or rebelliousness.

Imaginative portrayals of smoking, whether in canvases, photos, or films, add to the visual symbolism related with the training. Notorious pictures of film stars, performers, and social symbols smoking have become imbued in mainstream society, affecting view of smoking as exciting, defiant, or even optimistic. These social portrayals add to the social development of smoking as a way of behaving loaded down with representative importance.

Cultural impacts on smoking work at various levels, incorporating relational peculiarities, peer communications, financial variables, and the more extensive social milieu. The family, as the essential social unit, assumes a vital part in molding smoking ways of behaving. Kids frequently find out about smoking through perception of parental or familial smoking examples. Family mentalities toward smoking, whether lenient or prohibitive, fundamentally impact an individual's probability of starting and keeping on smoking.

Peer communications, particularly during pre-adulthood, significantly affect smoking commencement. The longing for social acknowledgment, peer pressure, and the impact of companions who smoke can add to the take-up of smoking among youthful people. The social setting where smoking happens — whether as a common action among companions or a defiant demonstration against cultural standards — assumes a significant part in forming the emotional experience of smoking.

Financial factors likewise add to the commonness and examples of smoking inside social orders. Smoking rates frequently display a financial inclination, with higher rates saw among people with lower pay and schooling levels.

The purposes behind this affiliation are intricate and complex, including variables, for example, designated advertising by the tobacco business, stressors related with lower financial status, and restricted admittance to smoking suspension assets.

The tobacco business' advertising procedures, by and large and in the current day, have taken advantage of social and cultural impacts to advance smoking. Ads frequently influence social images, way of life yearnings, and ideas of opportunity to make a positive picture around smoking. The relationship of smoking with ideas like insubordination, freedom, and refinement has been painstakingly developed to engage different segment gatherings.

Besides, the focusing of explicit social or subcultural bunches by the tobacco business has been an indisputable peculiarity. Networks with unmistakable social personalities, whether characterized by identity, age, or different variables, have been the focal point of custom-made promoting efforts. This designated approach intends to adjust smoking to social qualities, making a feeling of having a place or personality related with the utilization of tobacco items.

The standardization of smoking inside specific subcultures or groups of friends further builds up its social and cultural impact. In certain unique situations, smoking might be seen as a marker of adulthood, a method for adapting to pressure, or a method for mingling. These insights add to the entrenchment of smoking inside unambiguous social standards, making it trying to address through individual-centered mediations alone.

Government strategies and general wellbeing efforts assume a vital part in forming cultural perspectives toward smoking. Tobacco control measures, like tax assessment, sans smoke strategies, and realistic admonition names, can impact the social adequacy of smoking and add to changing social standards. Extensive tobacco control endeavors frequently include a mix of strategy, training, and local area based mediations to address the intricate transaction of social and cultural impacts.

The worldwide idea of the tobacco plague requires a familiarity with how social and cultural impacts work across various areas and networks. While smoking rates have declined in a major league salary nations because of viable tobacco control gauges, the commonness of smoking remaining parts high in some low- and center pay nations. Social and cultural elements, including the impact of global tobacco organizations, add to the diligence of smoking in these unique situations.

Endeavors to address social and cultural impacts on smoking ought to be socially delicate and setting explicit. Perceiving the variety of social standards and practices is fundamental for planning mediations that reverberate with explicit networks. Cooperation with local area pioneers, social powerhouses, and nearby associations can upgrade the adequacy of tobacco control endeavors by adjusting them to existing social qualities and needs.

All in all, the investigation of social and cultural effects on smoking uncovers the profoundly implanted nature of this conduct inside the texture of human social orders. From holy customs to famous media depictions, smoking has been woven into social practices and portrayals that shape individual decisions and cultural standards. Understanding and tending to these impacts is fundamental for creating far reaching and socially delicate tobacco control methodologies that go past individual way of behaving to handle the more extensive social elements that support the worldwide tobacco scourge.

## 2.3 The role of advertising and media in promoting smoking

The job of publicizing and media in advancing smoking is a complicated and compelling part of the tobacco plague. Since the beginning of time, the tobacco business has decisively utilized promoting and media missions to shape public discernments, make brand characters, and, at last, drive tobacco utilization. Understanding the components and strategies utilized by the tobacco business in publicizing and media is pivotal for creating viable general wellbeing intercessions and administrative measures to balance the effect of these limited time endeavors.

Promoting has for quite some time been perceived as an integral asset for impacting purchaser conduct, and the tobacco business has been a pioneer in using publicizing to make a positive picture around smoking. By and large, tobacco publicizing was inescapable across different media stations, including print, radio, and later, TV. The mid-twentieth century denoted a time of extreme tobacco publicizing, portrayed by notorious missions that formed the social scene and added to the standardization of smoking.

Print ads assumed a focal part in the early advancement of tobacco items. Notices included elaborate plans, enthralling symbolism, and powerful informing to connect smoking with helpful characteristics like complexity, fabulousness, and societal position. Tobacco organizations decisively adjusted their items to ideas of opportunity, freedom, and way of life goals, making a story that situated smoking as a basic piece of a beneficial way of life.

Magazines, papers, and announcements became materials for tobacco promoting imagination. Famous figures, for example, the Marlboro Man, a tough rancher, and the Joe Camel character, an adapted animation camel, became persevering through images of tobacco brands. These characters were painstakingly created to resound with explicit objective socioeconomics and make a brand personality that went past the actual item.

The coming of radio and, later, TV, carried new aspects to tobacco promoting. Radio projects and supported occasions flawlessly coordinated tobacco advancements, contacting a huge crowd. With the progress to TV, tobacco organizations gained by the visual medium to make important and genuinely resounding efforts. Cigarette plugs highlighting superstars, infectious jingles, and spectacular portrayals of smoking became ordinary during early evening TV.

The universality of tobacco promoting during this period significantly affected cultural standards and discernments. Smoking became inseparable from refinement, resistance, and an optimistic way of life. The consistent openness to positive portrayals of smoking in promoting added to the social acknowledgment and standardization of the way of behaving.

In light of developing worries about the wellbeing dangers of smoking, especially in the last part of the twentieth 100 years, the tobacco business confronted expanding examination and administrative difficulties. The milestone Top health spokesperson's Report in 1964 connecting smoking to cellular breakdown in the lungs denoted a defining moment in open mindfulness. Resulting administrative measures, for example, the prohibition on cigarette promoting on TV and radio in the US in 1971, planned to diminish the impact of tobacco publicizing on general wellbeing.

In any case, the tobacco business adjusted to these limitations by moving its publicizing techniques to different channels and embracing more unobtrusive methodologies. Print media, outside publicizing, and occasion sponsorships became conspicuous roads for tobacco advancements. The business additionally extended its span to worldwide business sectors, focusing on locales with less guidelines and different social settings.

The appearance of the web and advanced media in the late twentieth century gave new open doors and difficulties to tobacco promoting. Online stages became prolific ground for designated promoting, with tobacco organizations utilizing modern information examination to arrive at explicit socioeconomics. Online entertainment, specifically, turned into an integral asset for making brand networks, utilizing client produced content, and unpretentiously advancing smoking in manners that evaded customary promoting guidelines.

The idea of "marking" turned into a focal point of tobacco promoting systems. Brands were painstakingly created to summon explicit affiliations, ways of life, and feelings. The utilization of varieties, logos, and plan components meant to make a particular visual character for each brand, encouraging brand unwaveringness among purchasers. The bundling of tobacco items itself turned into a vehicle for publicizing, with particular plans and marking components building up the charm of explicit brands.

The idea of "light" or "low-tar" cigarettes arose as a showcasing methodology, it were a better choice to propose that these items. Regardless of proof running against the norm, these terms conveyed a feeling of diminished hurt, drawing in buyers worried about the wellbeing ramifications of smoking. The tobacco business effectively advanced the insight that these items were less destructive, adding to the confusion that they were a more secure choice.

Sponsorship of social and games turned into one more road for tobacco organizations to keep up with perceivability and advance their brands.

Equation 1 hustling, for example, had a well established relationship with tobacco sponsorships, with conspicuous brands embellished on race vehicles and related stock. The boundless openness created by such sponsorships built up the connection between tobacco brands and fervor, speed, and allure.

The tobacco business' impact reached out to item position in movies and TV programs, where smoking scenes were decisively embedded to build up the relationship among smoking and beneficial properties. Characters depicted as sure, defiant, or refined were many times portrayed smoking, further implanting the positive symbolism of smoking in mainstream society. The essential position of tobacco items inside the casing turned into an inconspicuous yet strong type of promoting.

The utilization of famous people as brand envoys likewise assumed a huge part in molding public view of smoking. Supports by entertainers, performers, and sports figures related smoking with popularity, achievement, and an insubordinate soul. The purposeful arrangement of big names with explicit tobacco brands made a powerful picture that resounded with fans and customers, further normalizing smoking according to people in general.

Lately, the tobacco business has adjusted to changing cultural perspectives and expanded consciousness of the wellbeing dangers of smoking. While customary types of publicizing keep on assuming a part, the center has moved to more current mediums, including web-based entertainment forces to be reckoned with and way of life marking. The utilization of powerhouses who advance tobacco items unpretentiously or by implication on stages like Instagram takes into consideration designated showcasing to explicit socioeconomics, frequently contacting more youthful crowds.

The rise of electronic cigarettes (e-cigarettes) and other novel nicotine conveyance items has presented new difficulties in managing tobacco promoting. The promoting of these items frequently accentuates subjects of damage decrease, way of life, and mechanical advancement. The utilization of flavors, smooth plan, and virtual entertainment powerhouses has added to the fame of these items, particularly among youth.

The effect of promoting and media on smoking stretches out past individual ways of behaving to impact cultural mentalities, social standards, and public arrangement. The unavoidable idea of tobacco promoting has added to the persevering through allure of smoking, in spite of many years of general wellbeing endeavors to control tobacco use. The business' capacity to adjust to administrative imperatives and influence advancing media scenes highlights the requirement for continuous carefulness and far reaching tobacco control measures.

General wellbeing efforts have looked to check the impact of tobacco promoting by giving counter-informing and underlining the wellbeing dangers of smoking.

Realistic admonition marks on cigarette bundling, hostile to smoking notices, and instructive drives have been utilized to bring issues to light and move cultural discernments. Nonetheless, the tobacco business' abundant resources and advertising aptitude keep on presenting difficulties to general wellbeing endeavors.

Administrative measures have been carried out to limit tobacco promoting and sponsorship in numerous nations. Prohibitions on tobacco publicizing in specific media, limitations right on track of-offer advancements, and plain bundling necessities are among the actions pointed toward diminishing the effect of promoting on smoking way of behaving. The viability of these actions shifts, and the tobacco business frequently looks for ways of dodging or challenge administrative limitations.

All in all, the job of publicizing and media in advancing smoking has been a strong power in forming social discernments, cultural standards, and individual ways of behaving. From the notorious missions of the mid-twentieth 100 years to the refined advanced procedures of the current day, the tobacco business has reliably utilized promoting to make positive relationship with smoking. The persevering through effect of these special endeavors highlights the requirement for thorough and versatile tobacco control procedures that address the complex idea of tobacco advancement across assorted media scenes.

The job of media in advancing smoking is a multi-layered and persuasive part of the more extensive tobacco pandemic. Media, enveloping a wide exhibit of stations like TV, radio, print, and, all the more as of late, computerized stages, plays had a critical impact in forming discernments, making social standards, and affecting individual ways of behaving connected with smoking. The complex connection among media and smoking traverses many years and mirrors the powerful development of the two enterprises.

By and large, print media filled in as an essential vehicle for tobacco publicizing, with papers and magazines highlighting elaborate missions that looked to connect smoking with positive credits. In the right on time to mid-twentieth hundred years, tobacco commercials were described by refined plans, reminiscent symbolism, and powerful informing. These missions meant to make a positive picture around smoking, connecting it with thoughts of excitement, complexity, and economic wellbeing.

The print medium took into account the formation of notable brand symbolism, with cigarette promotions frequently highlighting particular logos, colors, and slogans. The Marlboro Man, a rough cattle rustler, and the Joe Camel character, an adapted animation camel, are outstanding instances of notable figures that became inseparable from explicit tobacco brands. These pictures were painstakingly created to resound with target socioeconomics and make an enduring brand character.

Radio arose as a strong mechanism for tobacco promoting during the twentieth hundred years, permitting organizations to contact an expansive crowd through supported projects and jingles. Cigarette brands were frequently incorporated into well known public broadcasts, making relationship among smoking and diversion. The sound organization took into account the formation of essential jingles and expressions that further supported the positive symbolism of smoking.

The progress to TV denoted another period in tobacco publicizing, carrying both visual and hear-able aspects to limited time endeavors. Cigarette plugs turned into a staple of TV programming, including VIPs, infectious tunes, and fabulous portrayals of smoking. Brands looked to lay out close to home associations with watchers, connecting their items with subjects of opportunity, energy, and way of life goals.

TV publicizing arrived at remarkable degrees of omnipresence, adding to the standardization of smoking in regular daily existence. Smoking scenes became normal in famous TV programs and movies, with characters portrayed as certain, complex, and defiant frequently depicted as smokers. The intentional position of tobacco items inside scenes made unobtrusive yet effective relationship among smoking and helpful properties.

As worries about the wellbeing dangers of smoking developed, especially in the last 50% of the twentieth 100 years, administrative measures were executed to diminish tobacco promoting on TV and radio. The restriction on cigarette promoting on these stages in the US in 1971 denoted a huge achievement in general wellbeing endeavors to restrict the impact of media on smoking way of behaving.

Be that as it may, the tobacco business adjusted to these limitations by differentiating its promoting techniques and investigating elective media channels. Print media, open air publicizing, and sponsorships of social and games became noticeable roads for tobacco advancements. The development of the web and computerized media in the late twentieth century introduced new open doors and difficulties for tobacco publicizing.

The web worked with designated showcasing through internet based stages, permitting tobacco organizations to arrive at explicit socioeconomics with accuracy. Web-based entertainment, specifically, turned into a useful asset for making brand networks, utilizing client produced content, and unobtrusively advancing smoking in manners that bypassed conventional publicizing guidelines. Powerhouses, who frequently have huge followings on stages like Instagram and YouTube, became channels for advancing tobacco items by implication and contacting more youthful crowds.

The idea of "way of life marking" acquired noticeable quality in tobacco promoting, with brands situating themselves as images of specific ways of life and values.

This approach planned to make relationship among smoking and character, cultivating brand unwaveringness among shoppers. The tobacco business cautiously arranged internet based content that lined up with the brand's picture, frequently highlighting topics of defiance, opportunity, and independence.

Item situation in movies and network shows kept on being a strong type of tobacco promoting, with smoking scenes decisively embedded to build up the relationship among smoking and beneficial traits. The deliberate arrangement of tobacco brands with famous diversion properties made a strong subconscious effect on crowds, adding to the getting through allure of smoking.

The development of electronic cigarettes (e-cigarettes) and other novel nicotine conveyance items presented new difficulties in directing tobacco publicizing. E-cigarettes, advertised as options in contrast to customary cigarettes, frequently use advanced stages to advance their items. The business positions these items as mechanically progressed, smooth, and way of life situated, with flavors and plans that enticement for more youthful socioeconomics.

The effect of media in advancing smoking reaches out past promoting to the depiction of smoking in diversion content. While administrative measures have restricted unequivocal tobacco publicizing, the portrayal of smoking in movies and network shows stays a strong effect on cultural perspectives. Characters what smoke's identity is frequently depicted as certain, insubordinate, or modern, adding to the propagation of positive symbolism around smoking.

The tobacco business' effect on media isn't restricted to advancing customary tobacco items. It reaches out to the advancement of elective nicotine items, frequently outlined as damage decrease apparatuses. The business' capacity to adjust to developing media scenes and administrative conditions highlights the requirement for thorough and versatile tobacco control techniques.

Endeavors to balance the impact of media in advancing smoking have included general wellbeing efforts, strategy mediations, and instructive drives. Realistic admonition names on cigarette bundling, against smoking commercials, and instructive projects have looked to bring issues to light about the wellbeing dangers of smoking and check the positive symbolism sustained by media. Notwithstanding, the tobacco business' promoting ability and monetary assets present continuous difficulties to these endeavors.

Administrative measures have been carried out to confine tobacco promoting and sponsorship in numerous nations. Prohibitions on tobacco publicizing in specific media, limitations right on track of-offer advancements, and plain bundling necessities are among the actions pointed toward diminishing the effect of promoting on smoking way of behaving. Notwithstanding these endeavors, the worldwide idea of the tobacco business and the versatility of promoting systems require continuous watchfulness and composed global activity.

All in all, the job of media in advancing smoking has been a strong power in molding social discernments, cultural standards, and individual ways of behaving. From the notable publicizing efforts of the mid-twentieth hundred years to the complex advanced techniques of the current day, the tobacco business has reliably utilized media to make positive relationship with smoking. The getting through effect of these limited time endeavors highlights the requirement for complete and versatile tobacco control systems that address the multi-layered nature of media impact on smoking way of behaving.

# Chapter 3

### The Addictive Puzzle

In a world immersed with mechanical wonders and a consistent flood of data, the human psyche looks for shelter in different types of diversion. Among the heap decisions, there exists a particular and charming classification — the habit-forming puzzle. It is a domain where rationale and imagination merge, where the fulfillment of tackling a complicated conundrum entwines with the test of exploring through multifaceted labyrinths of thought.

At its center, the habit-forming puzzle is a complex element, including a different cluster of difficulties that range from the physical to the virtual, from the substantial to the theoretical. From old conundrums that have bewildered civic establishments for quite a long time to present day computerized puzzles that bridle the force of state of the art innovation, this type takes care of the intrinsic human craving to investigate, comprehend, and win.

One can't leave on a conversation about habit-forming puzzles without recognizing the significant effect they have had on mankind's set of experiences. The foundations of riddles can be followed back to old civic establishments where they served as a wellspring of diversion as well as instruments for instruction and mental activity.

The Sphinx's conundrum in Greek folklore, for example, exemplifies the combination of narrating and puzzle-settling, testing both keenness and mind.

As social orders advanced, so did the idea of riddles. They became implanted in different social works on, filling in as instruments for sending information, testing sharpness, and cultivating a feeling of local area. Whether it was the perplexing labyrinth plans of middle age houses of prayer or the emblematic riddles in Eastern way of thinking, mankind tracked down comfort in the specialty of mental investigation.

Quick forward to the contemporary period, and habit-forming puzzles have flawlessly incorporated into the texture of day to day existence. At this point not restricted to actual structures, they have tracked down another home in the advanced domain. Versatile applications and online stages offer an immense jungle gym for puzzle lovers, where the difficulties are basically as different as the actual players. Sudoku, crossword riddles, and jigsaw puzzles have become computerized friends, open with only a tap on a screen.

One of the captivating parts of habit-forming puzzles lies in their capacity to rise above generational limits. They have an immortal charm that spellbinds both the youthful and the old. Grandparents might find happiness in settling Sudoku puzzles in papers, while their grandkids submerge themselves in perplexing virtual getaway rooms. The riddle, it appears, has turned into an all inclusive language that opposes the limitations old enough and foundation.

The charm of habit-forming puzzles lies in their verifiable importance as well as in their ability to animate the brain. As the world plunges towards a time overwhelmed by innovation and robotization, the human mind longs for scholarly difficulties that go past the daily schedule. Puzzles, with their mind boggling designs and tricky arrangements, offer a safe house for mental investigation.

Take, for example, the cryptic universe of Rubik's Block — a three-layered puzzle that has bewildered and entranced personalities since its development during the 1970s. The block's dynamic tones and apparently vast stages disguise a complex algorithmic construction. Tackling it requires a mix of spatial thinking, design acknowledgment, and vital reasoning. The Rubik's 3D shape rises above its actual structure to turn into an image of tirelessness and scholarly victory.

In the computerized domain, puzzle games have advanced into refined encounters that push the limits of imagination and critical thinking. Games like Landmark Valley and The Observer present players with outwardly staggering scenes interweaved with puzzles that request a combination of imaginative appreciation and insightful reasoning. These advanced riddles rise above the conventional thoughts of ongoing interaction, offering vivid and contemplative excursions.

The habit-forming puzzle has likewise tracked down a sanctuary in the realm of math. Numerical riddles, with their exquisite straightforwardness and fundamental intricacy, draw in fans who revel in the excellence of numbers and rationale. From exemplary issues like the Monty Lobby difficulty to additional contemporary difficulties like the P versus NP issue, these riddles give a jungle gym to mathematicians and PC researchers to investigate the profundities of hypothetical thinking.

Past the domains of amusement and mental activity, habit-forming puzzles have secured themselves as strong instructive devices. Instructive riddles take special care of different age gatherings, presenting ideas in math, language, and science through intelligent and connecting with encounters. The gamification of learning has shown to be a compelling technique for encouraging interest and maintenance, obscuring the lines among schooling and diversion.

Be that as it may, the habit-forming nature of riddles accompanies its own arrangement of suggestions. Similarly as a spellbinding novel can consume hours of one's time, habit-forming puzzles can possibly obscure the limits among relaxation and fixation. The journey for tackling a difficult riddle can be all-consuming, driving people down a dark hole where time becomes slippery, and the rest of the world blurs out of spotlight.

In the time of moment satisfaction, where a universe of data lies readily available, habit-forming puzzles offer a relief from the steady torrent of improvements. They give an organized getaway, a psychological retreat where the current center strait to the prompt test. The charm of finishing a riddle takes advantage of the prize communities of the cerebrum, delivering a flood of dopamine that builds up the craving to proceed with the journey for arrangements.

However, this very appeal brings up issues about the barely recognizable difference between sound commitment and dependence. The expression "habit-forming puzzle" itself suggests a powerful mix of interest and impulse. While the larger part might enjoy puzzles as a type of recreation, there exists a subset for whom the pursuit turns into an unquenchable hankering, prompting a disregard of different parts of life.

In the domain of computerized puzzles, the reconciliation of social and serious components fuels the habit-forming potential. Online competitor lists, time sensitive difficulties, and multiplayer modes intensify the excitement of settling puzzles, transforming a lone movement into a collective encounter. The craving to beat friends and climb the positions adds a layer of seriousness that can change a relaxed side interest into a persistent pursuit.

Additionally, the approach of versatile gaming and the universality of cell phones have made habit-forming puzzles more open than any time in recent memory. The convenientce and comfort of these gadgets guarantee that a riddle is never in excess of a pocket away. The straightforwardness with which one can slip into the universe of riddles, whether during a drive or a snapshot of weariness, adds to their habit-forming nature.

The effect of habit-forming puzzles on emotional wellness is a subject of developing concern. While participating in riddles can upgrade mental capabilities and act as a pressure help system, over the top and impulsive riddle tackling may make unfavorable impacts. The line between a solid side interest and a fanatical way of behaving becomes obscured, bringing up issues about the possible outcomes on generally speaking prosperity.

Similarly as with any type of diversion or movement, control is critical. The habit-forming puzzle, when drawn nearer with a decent mentality, can be a wellspring of euphoria, scholarly feeling, and a method for cultivating strength despite challenges. It is the point at which the quest for puzzles rules one's time and thoughtfulness regarding the drawback of different parts of life that concerns emerge.

In the computerized age, where screens intervene our collaborations with the world, the habit-forming puzzle fills in as both a medicine and a likely entanglement. The test, then, at that point, lies in developing a careful way to deal with puzzle-tackling, where the advantages of mental feeling and delight are procured without capitulating to the alarm call of impulse.

The scene of habit-forming puzzles keeps on developing, molded by mechanical headways and the steadily changing elements of human way of behaving. Virtual and increased reality advancements vow to lift puzzle encounters higher than ever, obscuring the limits between the physical and the computerized. As these advances full grown, the vivid idea of riddles might additionally heighten their habit-forming request.

All in all, the habit-forming puzzle is a captivating crossing point of history, brain science, and innovation. From old enigmas that tried the insight of logicians to present day computerized difficulties that push the limits of innovativeness, puzzles have persevered as a demonstration of the human soul's journey for investigation and understanding. As we explore the unpredictable labyrinths of riddles in the advanced age, it is basic to move toward them with care, embracing the delight of tackling while at the same time defending against the traps of overabundance. The habit-forming puzzle, in its bunch structures, stays an enthralling conundrum — a wellspring of scholarly pleasure and, for some's purposes, an excursion with the potential for both illumination and snare.

## 3.1 Understanding the science behind nicotine addiction

Nicotine, a strong and exceptionally drug tracked down in tobacco items, has been a subject of extreme logical examination for a really long time. The comprehension of nicotine dependence includes disentangling the complicated exchange of neurobiology, brain science, and social factors that add to the turn of events and steadiness of this habit. This exhaustive investigation plans to dive into the science behind nicotine fixation, revealing insight into the systems that make it an imposing test for those endeavoring to stop.

At its center, nicotine enslavement is an intricate cycle that includes the mind's prize framework. Nicotine is the essential psychoactive substance in tobacco, applying its belongings by restricting to explicit receptors in the mind known as nicotinic acetylcholine receptors (nAChRs). These receptors are generally circulated all through the focal sensory system, assuming a significant part in different mental capabilities, including consideration, memory, and state of mind guideline.

At the point when nicotine is breathed in through smoking or different types of tobacco use, it quickly arrives at the mind, where it ties to nAChRs. This connection sets off the arrival of synapses, especially dopamine, which is a central member in the mind's prize circuit. Dopamine is related with sensations of delight and support, making a feeling of remuneration that turns out to be firmly connected to nicotine utilization.

The rehashed enactment of the prize framework by nicotine lays out a supporting circle. Over the long run, the cerebrum adjusts to the presence of nicotine by changing the awareness of its receptors and modifying the creation and arrival of synapses. These neuroadaptations add to the advancement of resilience, where higher dosages of nicotine are expected to accomplish similar pleasurable impacts.

As resistance creates, people might wind up expanding the recurrence and amount of nicotine utilization to keep up with the ideal degree of fulfillment. This heightening makes way for reliance, a sign of compulsion. Reliance is portrayed by the rise of withdrawal side effects when nicotine levels in the body decline. These side effects can go from peevishness and uneasiness to actual distress, making a strong motivating force to keep utilizing nicotine to mitigate these negative sensations.

The pattern of reliance turns out to be additionally settled in as people experience both physical and mental desires for nicotine. The mental part of dependence includes the affiliations framed between nicotine use and different prompts, like explicit conditions, exercises, or group environments. These signs can go about as strong triggers, evoking desires and supporting the constant idea of nicotine utilization.

Understanding the neurobiological underpinnings of nicotine enslavement gives an establishment to investigating the variables that add to its introduction and diligence. Hereditary elements assume a huge part in a singular's defenselessness to nicotine fixation. Varieties in qualities that encode for nicotinic receptors or compounds engaged with nicotine digestion can impact how an individual answers nicotine and their probability of creating reliance.

In addition, the age at which nicotine openness happens can affect weakness to enslavement. Puberty is a basic time of mental health, and openness to nicotine during this time can make enduring impacts. The creating mind is especially delicate to the remunerating properties of nicotine, and early openness can build the gamble of long haul dependence.

Social and ecological factors additionally add to the intricate scene of nicotine compulsion. Peer impact, social standards, and financial status can shape examples of tobacco use. The accessibility and openness of tobacco items, combined with showcasing and promoting systems, assume a urgent part in molding the social setting where nicotine use happens. Moreover, co-happening psychological wellness conditions, like melancholy or nervousness, can interface with nicotine fixation, making a mind boggling interaction of variables that add to its beginning and support.

Nicotine dependence isn't exclusively a result of individual decisions; it is profoundly interwoven with the more extensive cultural and ecological setting. Endeavors to address nicotine fixation require a complete comprehension of these complex impacts, recognizing that viable intercessions should stretch out past individual way of behaving to include social, monetary, and strategy aspects.

The excursion of nicotine enslavement, from commencement to reliance, includes an outpouring of neurochemical occasions inside the cerebrum. Unwinding this complicated web has prepared for the advancement of pharmacological intercessions pointed toward helping smoking end. Nicotine substitution treatments (NRTs), like patches, gum, and tablets, give controlled portions of nicotine to mitigate withdrawal side effects while continuously tightening the general nicotine admission. These treatments offer a damage decrease approach by isolating nicotine from the unsafe constituents of tobacco smoke.

Professionally prescribed meds, like bupropion and varenicline, target explicit synapse frameworks to lessen desires and withdrawal side effects. Bupropion, an abnormal upper, tweaks dopamine and norepinephrine levels in the mind, while varenicline goes about as a fractional agonist at nicotinic receptors, lessening the supporting impacts of nicotine.

While pharmacological mediations have shown viability in supporting smoking discontinuance, they are not panaceas. Achievement rates change, and backslide stays a typical test. Conduct mediations, for example, guiding and mental social treatment, assume a urgent part in tending to the mental parts of habit. These mediations assist people with creating survival techniques, distinguish sets off, and adjust standards of conduct related with nicotine use.

The scene of smoking end mediations is persistently developing, with arising advancements offering novel methodologies. Portable applications, computer generated reality programs, and online stages give available and customized apparatuses to help people in their quit endeavors. These innovations influence the standards of conduct science and mental rebuilding to improve inspiration and versatility during the difficult course of stopping smoking.

Notwithstanding, regardless of the accessibility of compelling intercessions, the excursion to smoking discontinuance is full of hindrances.

Nicotine fixation's strong hold on the mind, combined with the intricate interaction of hereditary, ecological, and mental elements, highlights the requirement for a complete and individualized way to deal with treatment. Perceiving that smoking suspension is definitely not a one-size-fits-all try is fundamental in fitting mediations to the remarkable requirements and difficulties looked by every person.

Besides, the cultural parts of nicotine compulsion require a more extensive viewpoint on counteraction and mischief decrease. General wellbeing efforts, administrative measures, and against tobacco arrangements add to establishing a climate less helpful for the inception and propagation of nicotine fixation. These endeavors, combined with designated instructive drives, plan to move accepted practices and lessen the predominance of tobacco use.

The coming of elective nicotine conveyance frameworks, like electronic cigarettes (e-cigarettes), has added a layer of intricacy to the scene of nicotine habit. While defenders contend that e-cigarettes offer a less hurtful option in contrast to customary burnable tobacco, concerns continue in regards to their security, particularly among youth. The allure of seasoned e-cigarettes, forceful showcasing, and the simple entry present difficulties to tobacco control endeavors, requiring continuous examination and administrative investigation.

The peculiarity of double use, where people at the same time utilize both customary tobacco items and e-cigarettes, further confounds the scene. Understanding the examples of double use and its suggestions for wellbeing results requires a nuanced approach that thinks about the remarkable qualities of every item and their consolidated effect on nicotine openness.

The logical investigation of nicotine fixation stretches out past the singular level to include populace wellbeing. Epidemiological examinations try to comprehend patterns in tobacco use, recognize risk factors, and assess the effect of mediations for a bigger scope. Reconnaissance frameworks, like public studies and wellbeing information bases, give important experiences into the commonness of tobacco use and examples of smoking way of behaving, directing general wellbeing methodologies and asset assignment.

While extensive headway has been made in disentangling the science behind nicotine habit, holes in information continue. The drawn out wellbeing impacts of arising tobacco and nicotine items, the effect of double use on wellbeing results, and the job of hereditary variables in treatment reaction are areas of continuous exploration. The powerful idea of the tobacco scene, with advancing items and promoting techniques, highlights the requirement for consistent logical request to illuminate proof based strategies and mediations.

All in all, understanding the science behind nicotine compulsion includes exploring a perplexing exchange of neurobiology, hereditary qualities, brain research, and cultural impacts. Nicotine's significant effect on the mind's award framework, combined with the unpredictable trap of elements that add to compulsion, highlights the difficulties looked by people endeavoring to stop smoking.

The diverse idea of nicotine habit requires a thorough and customized way to deal with treatment, coordinating pharmacological, conduct, and cultural mediations. Progressing logical exploration assumes a critical part in propelling comprehension we might interpret nicotine addiction.

### 3.2 Personal stories of addiction and attempts to quit

The accounts of dependence and endeavors to stop are profoundly private and changed, mirroring the exceptional excursions of people wrestling with the intricacies of substance use. These accounts epitomize the battles, wins, mishaps, and versatility that portray the difficult way towards recuperation. While every story is unmistakable, an ongoing idea winds through them — a faithful assurance to face the difficulties of dependence and fashion a way towards a better, sans substance life.

One such story rotates around Sarah, a youthful expert whose plummet into compulsion started harmlessly. At first trying different things with sporting medication use during school, Sarah wound up continuously trapped in a snare of reliance. What started as incidental utilize changed into a day to day custom, as substances turned into a survival technique for the burdens of work and individual life.

Sarah's acknowledgment of the profundity of her enslavement denoted the most vital phase in her excursion to recuperation. The affirmation that substances had taken command over her life provoked her to look for proficient assistance. This choice, nonetheless, was not without its obstacles. The disgrace related with compulsion and the apprehension about judgment constrained Sarah to wrestle with her battles peacefully for a drawn out period.

Ultimately, Sarah found comfort in a strong local area of people exploring comparative difficulties. Bunch treatment turned into a vital part of her recuperation, giving a place of refuge to share encounters, get direction, and cultivate a feeling of fellowship.

Sarah's process outlines the extraordinary force of local area support in breaking the disengagement that frequently goes with habit.

Conversely, Imprint's story reveals insight into the recurrent idea of fixation and backslide. Mark, a moderately aged father of two, had effectively beaten liquor enslavement in his twenties, just to end up entrapped by narcotic reliance in later years. A working environment injury prompted a remedy for pain relievers, accidentally starting a dangerous excursion into narcotic abuse.

Imprint's endeavors to stop were set apart by a progression of backslides, featuring the tenacious difficulties of breaking liberated from the grip of fixation. Each backslide filled in as an unmistakable sign of the considerable grasp substances can have on an individual, highlighting the requirement for far reaching and supported help in the recuperation cycle.

The job of relational peculiarities in enslavement and recuperation is exemplified in Maria's story. A mother of three, Maria's fight with liquor addiction was complicatedly laced with stressed familial connections. The effect of her habit resonated through her family, establishing a wild climate for her youngsters. The acknowledgment of the cost her habit was taking on her family filled in as an impetus for Maria's obligation to change.

Family-focused mediations and treatment assumed a urgent part in Maria's recuperation. Reconstructing trust, cultivating open correspondence, and tending to basic relational peculiarities became essential parts of her excursion towards collectedness. Maria's story features the interconnectedness of individual and familial prosperity with regards to dependence recuperation.

One more feature of the enslavement account is the exceptional difficulties looked by people engaging co-happening emotional well-being problems. Alex's story typifies this diversity, as he wrestled with both substance use and melancholy. The transaction between emotional well-being and enslavement represented an intricate arrangement of obstacles, requiring a coordinated and comprehensive way to deal with treatment.

Alex's process highlighted the significance of tending to fundamental emotional well-being issues with regards to fixation recuperation. Remedial modalities that enveloped both substance use and emotional wellness parts demonstrated instrumental in giving him the apparatuses to explore the unpredictable connection between the two.

The effect of natural elements on habit is discernibly portrayed in James' story. Experiencing childhood in an area overflowing with destitution and restricted open doors, James went to substance use as a survival strategy. The shortfall of positive good examples and restricted admittance to instructive and business possibilities established a favorable climate for the pattern of dependence on endure.

James' account reveals insight into the fundamental factors that add to the propagation of enslavement inside specific networks. It highlights the requirement for thorough intercessions that address individual battles as well as the more extensive financial determinants that fuel the pattern of substance misuse.

Every one of these individual stories highlights the multi-layered nature of enslavement and the significance of fitting intercessions to individual requirements. The variety of encounters features the requirement for a nuanced and compassionate methodology that considers the one of a kind difficulties looked by every person on their way to recuperation.

Endeavors to stop substance use are set apart by a range of techniques and intercessions, each intelligent of the singular's assets, emotionally supportive networks, and flexibility.

The customary model of compulsion treatment frequently includes a mix of detoxification, restoration, directing, and aftercare support. Notwithstanding, the viability of these intercessions changes, and the developing scene of dependence treatment consolidates inventive methodologies that perceive the powerful idea of substance use problems.

Pharmacotherapy has arisen as a foundation of habit treatment, offering meds that can relieve desires, mitigate withdrawal side effects, and deflect backslide. For people battling with narcotic fixation, drugs like methadone, buprenorphine, and naltrexone have shown viability in advancing restraint and supporting long haul recuperation. Essentially, drugs like disulfiram and acamprosate can support liquor end by instigating horrendous impacts upon liquor utilization.

While pharmacotherapy addresses the physiological parts of fixation, social mediations assume an essential part in tending to the mental and conduct parts. Mental conduct treatment (CBT), persuasive talking, and possibility the board are among the proof based remedial modalities that help people in understanding and changing maladaptive thought processes and conduct related with substance use.

The coming of computerized wellbeing advances has acquainted novel methodologies with compulsion treatment and recuperation support. Portable applications, computer generated reality programs, and online stages offer open and customized devices to people looking for help with their excursion towards restraint. These advancements influence the standards of conduct science, offering constant help, observing, and restorative intercessions.

Peer support has arisen as a strong part of enslavement recuperation, exemplified by shared help gatherings, for example, AA (AA) and Opiates Unknown (NA). The ethos of these gatherings spins around shared encounters, common consolation, and the confidence in the extraordinary force of local area. Peer support programs supplement formal treatment draws near, furnishing people with a feeling of having a place and understanding that rises above the clinical setting.

The job of otherworldliness and care in compulsion recuperation is exemplified in the story of Rachel. Battling with liquor compulsion, Rachel found comfort in an all encompassing methodology that coordinated otherworldly practices and care reflection into her recuperation process. The development of mindfulness, combined with an association with a higher reason, became fundamental to Rachel's capacity to conquer the difficulties presented by compulsion.

The variety of intercessions mirrors the acknowledgment that a one-size-fits-all way to deal with dependence treatment is insufficient. Individualized treatment designs that think about the exceptional requirements, inclinations, and difficulties of every individual are essential in encouraging effective results.

The developing scene of enslavement treatment ceaselessly integrates new modalities and creative methodologies, driven by a promise to improving the viability and openness of mediations.

In any case, the excursion towards recuperation isn't direct, and backslide stays a typical test. The stories of people who have encountered difficulties and backslides highlight the significance of review backslide as a part of the recuperation interaction as opposed to a disappointment. Understanding the triggers and factors adding to backslide can illuminate changes in accordance with treatment plans, supporting the strength and assurance of people on the way to recuperation.

The cultural viewpoint on compulsion is vital to molding public strategy, lessening shame, and encouraging a climate helpful for recuperation. The stories of people who have confronted judgment, separation, and seclusion because of their habit feature the inescapable shame related with substance use issues. Combatting shame requires a change in cultural perspectives, informed by sympathy, training, and a comprehension of the complicated variables that add to habit.

Regulative and strategy estimates assume a vital part in tending to the more extensive determinants of compulsion, from neediness and imbalance to admittance to medical care and training. Promotion for proof based arrangements, expanded subsidizing for habit treatment and counteraction programs, and the execution of mischief decrease procedures add to making a strong cultural structure for people looking for recuperation.

The individual accounts of compulsion and endeavors to stop enlighten the versatility of the human soul even with affliction. Every story is a demonstration of the limit with respect to change, development, and change. The affirmation that recuperation is a ceaseless, developing interaction highlights the requirement for progressing backing, understanding, and an aggregate obligation to tending .

### 3.3 The psychological aspects of smoking and dependency

The mental parts of smoking and reliance comprise a complicated exchange of mental, close to home, and conduct factors that add to the commencement, support, and difficulties related with stopping smoking. Understanding these mental aspects is urgent for creating viable intercessions and emotionally supportive networks that address the diverse idea of tobacco habit.

At the center of smoking's mental charm lies the perplexing connection between nicotine — the essential psychoactive substance in tobacco — and the cerebrum's award framework. Nicotine applies its belongings by restricting to nicotinic acetylcholine receptors in the mind, setting off the arrival of synapses like dopamine.

This neurochemical overflow makes sensations of joy and prize, laying out a building up circle that supports the relationship among smoking and positive feelings.

The mental reliance on smoking frequently appears as desires, a convincing craving to smoke that emerges in light of different prompts or triggers. These signals can be natural, social, or interior, including circumstances, feelings, or schedules related with smoking. The Pavlovian molding of these prompts with the pleasurable impacts of nicotine adds to the improvement of ongoing smoking examples.

Besides, smoking frequently fills in as a survival technique for stress, tension, or gloomy feelings. The demonstration of smoking becomes entwined with profound guideline, offering a flashing getaway or interruption from life's difficulties. This close to home reliance on smoking convolutes the method involved with stopping, as people might fear losing an apparent wellspring of solace or stress help.

The mental parts of smoking are likewise unpredictably connected to the idea of self-personality. For some people, smoking becomes weaved with their healthy identity, impacting how they see and present themselves to other people. The ceremonial idea of smoking, from the demonstration of lighting a cigarette to the social parts of smoking in gatherings, adds to the development of a smoking personality that can be profoundly imbued.

The social component of smoking further emphasizes its mental effect. Smoking is much of the time a shared movement, making a feeling of having a place and kinship among smokers. The common experience of smoking in group environments builds up the mental bonds conformed to tobacco use, making stopping an individual test as well as a social one.

The mental parts of smoking reach out past the actual demonstration to the expectation of smoking and the apparent advantages related with it. The expectation of the pleasurable impacts of nicotine, combined with the adapted reaction to smoking prompts, intensifies the mental support that supports the propensity. Breaking this support circle is a basic part of smoking suspension endeavors, requiring a designated center around both the mental and conduct aspects of reliance.

Endeavors to stop smoking frequently experience the mental peculiarity of withdrawal, which incorporates a scope of side effects as the body changes with the shortfall of nicotine. These side effects incorporate touchiness, nervousness, trouble concentrating, and profound desires. The mental pain related with withdrawal represents a huge hindrance to stopping and highlights the requirement for thorough help during the end cycle.

The brain science of smoking is additionally impacted by the idea of seen control. People might persuade themselves that they have command over their smoking propensities, permitting them to legitimize proceeded with tobacco use.

This impression of control, frequently energized by the irregular support of pleasurable smoking encounters, can block the acknowledgment of the developing reliance on nicotine.

The job of mental cycles in smoking is obvious in the peculiarity of mental discord, where people experience mental distress when their convictions or perspectives struggle with their way of behaving. Smokers might wrestle with the attention to the wellbeing gambles related with smoking while at the same time proceeding with the propensity. Settling mental discord is a basic move toward the excursion towards stopping, requiring a change in mental structures and conviction frameworks.

The mental parts of smoking are not static; they develop over the long haul and are impacted by different life stages, stressors, and ecological elements. Puberty, specifically, is a weak period for the commencement of smoking, as people explore personality development, peer impact, and a longing for independence. The interaction of formative variables and mental weaknesses during this stage highlights the significance of designated counteraction endeavors.

Pregnancy acquaints one more aspect with the mental parts of smoking, as maternal worries for fetal wellbeing meet with the difficulties of nicotine reliance. The inspiration to safeguard the unborn youngster can act as a strong impetus for smoking discontinuance, featuring the powerful exchange between mental elements and the changing setting of life altering situations.

Understanding the mental components of smoking is vital for planning powerful intercessions that address the underlying drivers of reliance. Conduct treatments, like mental social treatment (CBT), center around distinguishing and adjusting the maladaptive idea examples and ways of behaving related with smoking. These intercessions furnish people with survival methods, stress the executives procedures, and mental rebuilding abilities to explore the difficulties of stopping.

Persuasive meeting, one more restorative methodology, looks to upgrade a person's natural inspiration to stop smoking by investigating and settling indecision. By taking part in unassuming discussions and directing people to explain their purposes behind change, persuasive meeting tends to the mental irresoluteness that frequently goes with endeavors to stop.

The joining of care based mediations into smoking end programs addresses a developing pattern in tending to the mental parts of dependence. Care rehearses, like care contemplation and careful smoking, underline present-second mindfulness and non-critical acknowledgment. These procedures can upgrade self-guideline, lessen incautious ways of behaving, and give people an uplifted consciousness of their smoking triggers.

The appearance of computerized wellbeing advances has presented imaginative instruments that influence mental standards to help smoking end.

Portable applications, for instance, utilize conduct science techniques, following advancement, sending updates, and giving fitted input to upgrade inspiration and adherence to stop plans. Computer generated reality programs submerge people in recreated conditions that imitate smoking prompts, offering a controlled setting for openness treatment and desensitization.

The brain science of smoking suspension is additionally impacted by the idea of backslide and the elements that add to the repeat of smoking after a quit endeavor. Backslide is many times conceptualized as an interaction as opposed to an occasion, including a few phases, including profound backslide, mental backslide, and actual backslide. Perceiving the signs and triggers of backslide at each stage is pivotal for carrying out opportune intercessions.

Social help assumes a vital part in the mental scene of smoking suspension. The consolation, understanding, and support given by companions, family, and care groups can altogether influence a singular's inspiration and capacity to stop smoking. The common experience of stopping inside a strong local area can relieve sensations of confinement and cultivate a feeling of aggregate versatility.

The mental parts of smoking end are likewise affected by the more extensive social and cultural setting. Hostile to smoking efforts, strategy measures, and changes in accepted practices add to changing the aggregate view of smoking. The denormalization of smoking inside society, combined with expanded attention to the wellbeing chances, changes the mental scene encompassing tobacco use and builds up the inspiration to stop.

In addition, financial elements, like the expense of tobacco items and admittance to medical care, impact the brain research of smoking. Monetary contemplations, joined with the rising cultural attention to the financial weight of tobacco-related ailments, add to the inspiration for smoking suspension and strategy support.

All in all, the mental parts of smoking and reliance are many-sided, enveloping a range of mental, close to home, and social elements. The interlaced connection among nicotine and the mind's prize framework, combined with the molding of smoking prompts, shapes the underpinning of mental reliance. Mediations that focus on these mental aspects, including conduct treatments, care rehearses, and computerized wellbeing instruments, offer an exhaustive way to deal with smoking discontinuance.

The mental scene of smoking is dynamic, advancing after some time and impacted by different life stages, stressors, and ecological variables. Pre-adulthood and pregnancy present interesting difficulties, accentuating the requirement for designated avoidance and suspension endeavors during these basic periods. The coordination of social help, social movements, and monetary contemplations further shapes the brain science of smoking suspension, adding to the continuous change of cultural perspectives towards tobacco use.

Smoking and reliance comprise a diverse issue with significant ramifications for general wellbeing. The demonstration of smoking, essentially connected with the utilization of tobacco, has developed from social ceremonies to a worldwide wellbeing concern. Understanding the interaction between the physiological and mental parts of smoking is urgent for fathoming the intricacies of reliance and planning powerful systems for discontinuance.

Physiologically, the habit-forming nature of smoking is firmly connected to nicotine, a normally happening alkaloid found in tobacco leaves. Nicotine goes about as the central psychoactive part answerable for the building up impacts of smoking. When breathed in, nicotine quickly crosses the blood-cerebrum obstruction and ties to nicotinic acetylcholine receptors in the mind, prompting the arrival of synapses, most quite dopamine.

Dopamine, frequently alluded to as the "vibe great" synapse, assumes a focal part in the cerebrum's prize framework. The flood of dopamine initiated by nicotine causes pleasurable situations and a feeling of remuneration, building up the relationship among smoking and good encounters. This neurobiological component underlies the underlying fascination with smoking and contributes altogether to the advancement of reliance.

The course of reliance unfurls as rehashed openness to nicotine prompts neuro-adaptations inside the mind. The cerebrum changes with the presence of nicotine by expanding the number and responsiveness of nicotinic receptors. This peculiarity, known as upregulation, brings about an increased reaction to nicotine, expecting people to consume more to accomplish similar pleasurable impacts — an event ordinarily alluded to as resilience.

Resistance makes way for expanded nicotine utilization, encouraging a pattern of heightening use. In addition, the withdrawal of nicotine, described by side effects like crabbiness, nervousness, and desires, results when levels of the substance decrease in the body. The aversive idea of withdrawal makes a strong motivating force to keep smoking, propagating the pattern of reliance.

The physiological parts of smoking and nicotine reliance are additionally confounded by the strategy for conveyance. Inward breath, through smoking or vaping, gives a fast course to nicotine ingestion, heightening its belongings. The demonstration of smoking turns out to be unpredictably connected with the pharmacological impacts of nicotine, making a ceremonial way of behaving that adds to the mental components of reliance.

Past the physiological domain, the mental parts of smoking assume a crucial part in supporting the propensity. The ceremonial idea of smoking — lighting a cigarette, enjoying conscious drags, and encountering the tangible parts of smoke inward breath — inserts the conduct inside everyday schedules and exercises. These ceremonies become interlaced with different parts of life, like mingling, stress help, or snapshots of thought.

The mental appeal of smoking is complicatedly attached to its relationship with social and social settings. Smoking has generally been implanted in customs, services, and get-togethers, forming its discernment as a public movement. The common experience of smoking encourages a feeling of brotherhood and having a place, adding to the social support of the way of behaving.

Social standards and cultural perspectives towards smoking further impact its mental aspects. In certain societies, smoking might be seen as a soul changing experience or an image of development, supporting its enticement for specific socioeconomics. On the other hand, hostile to smoking efforts and changes in cultural discernments have looked to check these standards, expecting to denormalize smoking and decrease its social adequacy.

The mental parts of smoking reach out to the domain of self-character. For some people, smoking becomes woven into their healthy identity, affecting how they see and present themselves. Smokers might connect smoking with characteristics like unwinding, refinement, or disobedience, developing a smoking personality that adds to the obstruction of stopping.

Reliance on smoking is frequently entwined with survival techniques for stress, tension, or pessimistic feelings. The demonstration of smoking gives a transient getaway, a ritualized stop that permits people to explore the intricacies of life. Smoking turns into a self-mitigating component, making a mental reliance on the way of behaving for the purpose of profound guideline.

The mental components of smoking reach out to the expectant delight related with the demonstration. The simple expectation of smoking and the apparent advantages connected to it add to the building up circle that supports the propensity. This part of anticipation, combined with the adapted reaction to smoking prompts, enhances the mental support that ties the way of behaving.

Tending to the intricacies of smoking and reliance requires a thorough comprehension of both the physiological and mental parts. Smoking suspension endeavors frequently include a mix of pharmacological intercessions and conduct treatments. Nicotine substitution treatments (NRTs), like patches, gum, and tablets, give controlled dosages of nicotine to ease withdrawal side effects while steadily diminishing by and large nicotine admission.

Pharmacotherapies, for example, doctor prescribed prescriptions like bupropion and varenicline, target synapse frameworks to diminish desires and withdrawal side effects. While these prescriptions address the physiological parts of reliance, conduct treatments dig into the mental aspects, expressing methodologies to adjust impression designs, adapt to triggers, and develop versatility during the end interaction.

Social treatments, like mental conduct treatment (CBT) and possibility the board, assume an essential part in smoking end. CBT centers around recognizing and changing maladaptive idea examples and ways of behaving related with smoking. By tending to mental bends and giving adapting abilities, CBT outfits people with the apparatuses to explore the mental difficulties of stopping.

Possibility the board, then again, utilizes a support based approach. Uplifting feedback, as remunerations or motivating forces, is utilized to urge forbearance and adherence to stop plans. This conduct mediation use standards of operant molding to reinforce wanted ways of behaving, giving substantial motivators to accomplishing smoking suspension achievements.

The approach of advanced wellbeing advances has acquainted creative apparatuses with help smoking suspension endeavors. Portable applications, augmented reality programs, and online stages influence mental standards to upgrade inspiration and adherence to stop plans. These advances offer constant help, checking, and restorative intercessions, taking care of the assorted requirements of people trying to stop smoking.

Care based mediations address a developing pattern in tending to the mental parts of smoking. Care rehearses, like care contemplation and careful smoking, underline present-second mindfulness and non-critical acknowledgment. These procedures upgrade self-guideline, lessen hasty ways of behaving, and uplift familiarity with smoking triggers, encouraging a careful way to deal with the end interaction.

Peer backing and gathering mediations comprise a fundamental component in tending to the social and mental elements of smoking. Smoking discontinuance support gatherings, both face to face and on the web, furnish people with a feeling of local area, shared encounters, and common consolation. The aggregate strength of a strong gathering can moderate sensations of seclusion and build up the mental determination required for effective stopping.

The mental parts of smoking are not segregated to the individual; they reach out to the more extensive cultural and social setting. Hostile to smoking efforts, strategy measures, and changes in accepted practices add to changing impression of smoking. The denormalization of smoking inside society, combined with expanded attention to the wellbeing gambles, changes the mental scene encompassing tobacco use and builds up the inspiration to stop.

Financial contemplations, like the expense of tobacco items and admittance to medical services, further impact the brain research of smoking. Monetary worries, combined with the rising cultural consciousness of the financial weight of tobacco-related diseases, add to the inspiration for smoking suspension and promotion for strategy measures pointed toward decreasing smoking commonness.

Taking everything into account, the intricate interaction of physiological and mental elements underlies smoking and reliance. Nicotine's effect on the cerebrum's prize framework makes an intense building up circle, adding to the turn of events and support of reliance. The mental components of smoking, from formal ways of behaving to social and social affiliations, intensify the difficulties related with stopping.

Exhaustive smoking suspension systems perceive the need to address both the physiological and mental parts of reliance. Pharmacological mediations, conduct treatments, care rehearses, computerized wellbeing instruments, and companion support by and large add to a comprehensive methodology that recognizes the multi-layered nature of smoking and furnishes people with the devices and backing required for fruitful end. Understanding the mind boggling connection between the physiological and mental components of smoking is fundamental for creating compelling intercessions and encouraging a sans smoke future.

# Chapter 4

### Smoke and Mirrors – The Tobacco Industry's Secrets

Tobacco, a plant local to the Americas, has a long and questionable history. For a really long time, native people groups involved tobacco for profound and therapeutic purposes. In any case, with the appearance of Europeans in the Americas, tobacco took an alternate direction. It turned into a worthwhile ware, developed and exchanged on a worldwide scale. The tobacco business, as far as we might be concerned today, has profound roots in this mind boggling history, and with its ascent came financial success as well as a foreboding shadow of mysteries and control.

The twentieth century saw the fast industrialization and commercialization of the tobacco business. Cigarette smoking, specifically, turned into a far reaching social peculiarity, glamorized by promoting and Hollywood. Notwithstanding, in the background, the business was covering vital data about the wellbeing chances related with tobacco use.

Logical proof connecting smoking to cellular breakdown in the lungs and other serious ailments started to arise during the twentieth hundred years. Specialists like Richard Doll and A. Bradford Slope led milestone concentrates on that laid out a reasonable association among smoking and cellular breakdown in the lungs. The discoveries sent shockwaves through the clinical local area, yet the tobacco business answered with a mission of refusal and confusion.

Inside records later uncovered an upsetting example of misdirection inside the business. Tobacco organizations knew about the wellbeing takes a chance with presented by their items, yet they effectively attempted to stifle this data and cast uncertainty on logical examination. The expression "purposeful misdirection" took on another importance as the business participated in a conscious mission to make disarray and plant seeds of uncertainty among people in general.

One of the most scandalous cases of this control was the business' endeavors to minimize the habit-forming nature of nicotine. Inside notices from significant tobacco organizations, like Philip Morris and RJ Reynolds, showed a determined procedure to control nicotine levels in cigarettes to improve dependence. The objective was to keep smokers snared and guarantee a constant flow of income, all while denying any purposeful endeavors to make cigarettes more habit-forming.

Advertising assumed a significant part in the tobacco business' mission of trickery. Promotions depicted smoking as stylish and complex, partner it with progress and social acknowledgment. Big names were in many cases highlighted in these missions, making a deception of an association among smoking and a beneficial way of life. The Marlboro Man, a rough rancher frequently portrayed riding a horse, turned into a notable image of this promoting technique.

The business additionally designated explicit socioeconomics, like ladies and youngsters, with custom-made promoting efforts. Ladies were promoted cigarettes as an image of freedom and strengthening, while the tobacco business decisively situated itself as an ally of ladies' privileges. In the mean time, commercials outfitted towards the adolescent depicted smoking as a demonstration of resistance and opportunity.

Away from public scrutiny, nonetheless, tobacco leaders were completely mindful of the damage their items were causing. In 1994, seven Presidents from significant tobacco organizations affirmed before the US Congress, recognizing that nicotine was habit-forming and that smoking caused different illnesses, including cellular breakdown in the lungs. This turning point denoted a defining moment in open discernment, however the business kept on battling against administrative measures.

Fights in court resulted, with tobacco organizations confronting claims from people and states looking for remuneration for the wellbeing costs related with smoking. The Expert Settlement Understanding in 1998 was a milestone lawful settlement between significant tobacco organizations and 46 U.S. states.

The settlement planned to recuperate medical services costs brought about by states because of smoking-related ailments and forced limitations on tobacco promoting.

Regardless of these legitimate difficulties, the tobacco business proceeded to adjust and develop. The development of e-cigarettes and other elective nicotine conveyance frameworks introduced new open doors for the business to keep up with its grasp on purchasers. While promoted as a less hurtful option in contrast to customary cigarettes, these items raised worries about their own wellbeing chances and their capability to draw in another age of nicotine clients.

Lately, the vaping business, overwhelmed by organizations like Juul, confronted examination for its job in the adolescent vaping pestilence. The smooth and tactful plan of e-cigarettes, alongside tempting flavors, spoke to a more youthful segment. The flood in vaping among youths raised alerts, provoking administrative activities and examinations concerning the advertising practices of these organizations.

The tobacco business' privileged insights reached out past wellbeing related issues. Reports uncovered a long history of political impact and impedance in open strategy. Campaigning endeavors, crusade commitments, and key partnerships with political figures permitted the business to shape regulation and administrative systems in support of its. The rotating entryway between the tobacco business and government organizations raised worries about irreconcilable circumstances and compromised general wellbeing drives.

Worldwide components of the tobacco business' impact were likewise apparent. Agricultural nations became landmarks for tobacco organizations looking for new business sectors as smoking rates declined in the Western world. Forceful showcasing strategies designated weak populaces, and remiss guidelines in certain locales permitted the business to work with relative exemption.

One outstanding model was the business' resistance to tobacco control estimates proposed by the World Wellbeing Association (WHO). The Structure Show on Tobacco Control (FCTC), a worldwide general wellbeing settlement, planned to address the global elements of tobacco control. Be that as it may, the tobacco business effectively campaigned against the FCTC and tried to subvert its arrangements.

Corporate social obligation (CSR) drives arose as one more device in the tobacco business' munitions stockpile. By financing widespread developments, instructive projects, and admirable missions, tobacco organizations endeavored to depict themselves as mindful corporate residents. This methodology intended to counter bad insights and fabricate unions with powerful partners.

Notwithstanding these endeavors, public consciousness of the business' strategies kept on developing. Narratives, analytical news-casting, and promotion crusades uncovered the dull underside of the tobacco business, prompting expanded public tension for stricter guidelines and responsibility.

The coming of virtual entertainment further enhanced the voices of hostile to tobacco advocates and gave a stage to sharing data about the business' practices. Online people group mobilized against the control strategies utilized by tobacco organizations, encouraging a worldwide development for tobacco control and general wellbeing.

Tobacco control strategies, including expanded tax assessment, realistic admonition names, and smoking boycotts, built up some decent forward momentum in numerous nations. These actions intended to lessen tobacco utilization, safeguard general wellbeing, and moderate the financial weight of smoking-related diseases on medical services frameworks.

The battle against the tobacco business' mysteries likewise stretched out to the domain of logical exploration. Autonomous examinations and examinations kept on uncovering new elements of the business' strategies, revealing insight into already undisclosed data. Specialists confronted difficulties, including industry-supported investigations intended to make disarray and subvert the believability of against tobacco research.

The fight for straightforwardness and responsibility in the tobacco business stays continuous. While progress has been made in bringing issues to light and carrying out tobacco control measures, challenges continue. The business' capacity to adjust to evolving conditions, combined with its impressive monetary assets, represents a consistent danger to general wellbeing drives.

Endeavors to uncover the tobacco business' mysteries should stay watchful and complex. Fortifying guidelines, supporting free examination, and encouraging worldwide cooperation are fundamental parts of an exhaustive technique to defy the business' underhanded practices. Public mindfulness and schooling assume an essential part in engaging people to settle on informed decisions about tobacco use and in considering the business responsible for its activities.

All in all, the tobacco business' mysteries structure a dull embroidery of misdirection, control, and double-dealing. From the beginning of cigarette promoting to the contemporary difficulties presented by e-cigarettes, the business has reliably focused on benefits over general wellbeing. Unwinding the deliberate misdirection requires an aggregate exertion from legislatures, common society, and people to uncover reality, execute powerful guidelines, and protect general wellbeing from the deceptive impact of the tobacco business.

**4.1 Unveiling the tactics used by the tobacco industry**

Tobacco, a plant with profound roots in the Americas, plays had a huge impact in molding the direction of mankind's set of experiences. From its stylized and therapeutic use among native people groups to its change into a worldwide ware, tobacco's process has been both unpredictable and disputable. In any case, behind the shroud of the tobacco business' financial achievement lies a mind boggling snare of strategies, trickery, and control that have had significant outcomes on general wellbeing and society.

The rise of the tobacco business in the twentieth century denoted a defining moment in the connection among people and this plant. As cigarettes acquired fame, so did the business' endeavors to hide basic data about the wellbeing gambles related with smoking. Logical proof connecting smoking to cellular breakdown in the lungs and different illnesses started to surface, because of spearheading specialists like Richard Doll and A. Bradford Slope. Their work set up for a conflict between general wellbeing and corporate interests that would characterize the a long time to come.

Inward records later uncovered a stunning truth: significant tobacco organizations were very much aware of the risks presented by their items. Notwithstanding this information, they participated in a determined mission to stifle data and cast uncertainty on logical examination. This intentional demonstration of misdirection became known as the business' utilization of "purposeful misdirection," an illustration for making disarray and darkening reality with regards to the risks of smoking.

At the core of the tobacco business' plots was the purposeful control of nicotine levels in cigarettes. Inner notices from organizations like Philip Morris and RJ Reynolds uncovered an essential work to upgrade the habit-forming properties of cigarettes. The objective was clear — to keep shoppers snared and guarantee a persistent progression of benefits. While leaders openly denied any purposeful endeavors to increment compulsion, their interior correspondences laid out an alternate picture, uncovering an unfeeling negligence for the wellbeing and prosperity of their clients.

Advertising assumed a vital part in the tobacco business' mission of duplicity.

Notices glamorized smoking, partner it with progress, refinement, and even resistance. The Marlboro Man, a notorious figure depicted as a rough rancher, turned into an image of the business' promoting ability. Superstars were enrolled to embrace cigarettes, making a deception of fabulousness and attractiveness. In the mean time, in secret, the business kept on smothering data about the dangers related with smoking.

Ladies turned into a particular objective for tobacco promoting, with crusades intended to connect smoking with freedom and strengthening. The business decisively situated itself as an ally of ladies' privileges, all while disregarding the unfavorable wellbeing impacts of smoking on ladies. Youngsters, as well, were not saved from the business' strategies. Commercials focused on the young depicted smoking as a demonstration of disobedience and opportunity, making a perilous charm that would have expansive outcomes.

The business' guile arrived at a limit in 1994 when seven Presidents from significant tobacco organizations affirmed before the US Congress. Having sworn to tell the truth, they conceded that nicotine was habit-forming and that smoking caused different infections, including cellular breakdown in the lungs. This turning point ought to have denoted a defining moment, yet the tobacco business kept on opposing significant change and administrative measures.

Fights in court resulted, with tobacco organizations confronting claims from people and legislatures looking for remuneration for the wellbeing costs related with smoking. The Expert Settlement Understanding in 1998 was a huge turn of events, driving significant tobacco organizations to pay billions of dollars to 46 U.S. states to take care of medical services costs connected with smoking-related ailments. The settlement likewise forced limitations on tobacco advertising, however the business' flexibility permitted it to investigate new roads for keeping up with its impact.

The ascent of elective nicotine conveyance frameworks, like e-cigarettes, gave the tobacco business another open door. Promoted as a less hurtful option in contrast to conventional cigarettes, these items raised worries about their own wellbeing chances and their capability to draw in another age of nicotine clients. The business' capacity to turn and adjust to changing conditions highlighted its flexibility and assurance to get its spot on the lookout.

The vaping business, overwhelmed by organizations like Juul, confronted its own arrangement of discussions. The smooth plan and tempting kinds of e-cigarettes spoke to a more youthful segment, prompting a flood in vaping among young people. Administrative activities and examinations were started to address the promoting practices of these organizations and their part in the adolescent vaping plague. Yet again the business' strategies of speaking to a more youthful crowd brought up moral issues and reestablished calls for severe guidelines.

The tobacco business' mysteries reached out past wellbeing related issues. Records uncovered a long history of political impact and obstruction in open strategy. Through campaigning endeavors, crusade commitments, and key coalitions with political figures, the business formed regulation and administrative structures in support of its.

The spinning entryway between the tobacco business and government organizations raised worries about irreconcilable circumstances, risking general wellbeing drives and putting the business' advantages in front of the prosperity of the populace.

On the global stage, the tobacco business' impact was apparent in its forceful venture into non-industrial nations. As smoking rates declined in the Western world, these areas became milestones for the business looking for new business sectors. Forceful promoting strategies designated weak populaces, and careless guidelines permitted the business to work with relative exemption. The worldwide idea of the business' tasks made it moving for individual nations to go up against and direct really.

Resistance to worldwide tobacco control estimates proposed by the World Wellbeing Association (WHO) featured the business' assurance to safeguard its inclinations. The Structure Show on Tobacco Control (FCTC), a worldwide general wellbeing deal, confronted furious opposition from the tobacco business. Campaigning endeavors and endeavors to subvert the FCTC's arrangements displayed the business' negligence for global endeavors to control tobacco utilization and safeguard general wellbeing.

Corporate social obligation (CSR) drives arose as an essential instrument for the tobacco business to counter bad insights. By subsidizing far-reaching developments, instructive projects, and worthy missions, tobacco organizations looked to introduce themselves as dependable corporate residents. This determined exertion planned to divert consideration from the business' unsafe practices and assemble partnerships with compelling partners.

Notwithstanding these endeavors at picture restoration, public consciousness of the business' strategies kept on developing. Narratives, insightful reporting, and promotion crusades uncovered the dim underside of the tobacco business, prompting expanded public strain for stricter guidelines and responsibility. The force of virtual entertainment assumed a vital part in enhancing the voices of hostile to tobacco advocates, giving a stage to sharing data and coordinating a worldwide development for tobacco control and general wellbeing.

Tobacco control arrangements picked up speed because of public mindfulness and backing endeavors. Expanded tax assessment, realistic admonition names, and smoking boycotts were among the actions carried out to diminish tobacco utilization, safeguard general wellbeing, and reduce the monetary weight of smoking-related ailments on medical services frameworks.

The fight for straightforwardness and responsibility in the tobacco business stretched out to the domain of logical examination. Autonomous examinations and examinations kept on uncovering new components of the business' strategies, revealing insight into already undisclosed data. Analysts confronted difficulties, including industry-financed investigations intended to make disarray and sabotage the validity of against tobacco research. The requirement for thorough, fair examination turned out to be progressively basic in countering the business' endeavors to control public discernment.

Endeavors to uncover the tobacco business' mysteries should stay cautious and diverse. Reinforcing guidelines, supporting free examination, and encouraging worldwide coordinated effort are fundamental parts of an exhaustive methodology to stand up to the business' underhanded practices. Public mindfulness and schooling assume an essential part in engaging people to settle on informed decisions about tobacco use and in considering the business responsible for its activities.

All in all, divulging the strategies utilized by the tobacco business uncovers an upsetting story of double dealing, control, and abuse. From the conscious disguise of wellbeing dangers to the vital focusing of explicit socioeconomics, the business' activities have had extensive results. While progress has been made in bringing issues to light and carrying out tobacco control measures, challenges endure. The tobacco business' flexibility and monetary assets represent a steady danger to general wellbeing drives. Exposing the deliberate misdirection requires a continuous obligation to straightforwardness, responsibility, and an aggregate work to safeguard the prosperity of people and networks all over the planet.

### 4.2 Exposé on marketing strategies targeting vulnerable populations

The universe of showcasing is a dynamic and persuasive power that shapes shopper conduct, impacts decisions, and frequently reflects cultural qualities. Notwithstanding, a hazier side of promoting arises when certain ventures intentionally target weak populaces for their own benefit. In this confession, we dig into the tricky methodologies utilized by different enterprises, especially the tobacco business, as they exploit and control weak gatherings, putting benefit before the prosperity of people and networks.

The tobacco business, with its long and disagreeable history, has been an infamous professional of focusing on weak populaces. Quite possibly of the most powerless and intensely designated bunch has been ladies. Throughout the long term, the business decisively created promoting efforts pointed toward partner smoking with ideas of autonomy, strengthening, and complexity for ladies. Cigarette promotions frequently portrayed fabulous ladies, connecting smoking to a freed and current way of life. The utilization of trademarks like "You've made some amazing progress, child" with regards to ladies smoking additionally highlighted the business' endeavor to adjust smoking to the women's activist development.

Behind this façade of strengthening, in any case, lay a more obscure reality. The tobacco business' showcasing strategies towards ladies helpfully disregarded the deep rooted wellbeing gambles related with smoking, including an elevated gamble of cellular breakdown in the lungs and different illnesses. While ladies were persuaded to think that smoking was an image of freedom, the business unfeelingly dismissed the likely ramifications for their wellbeing.

Youngsters, as well, have been a practical objective for the tobacco business' promoting hardware. Perceiving the pliability of youth culture and the craving for disobedience, the business has reliably depicted smoking as a demonstration of rebellion and autonomy. Ads frequently highlighted energetic and lighthearted pictures, partner smoking with experience and defiance to cultural standards.

The utilization of energetic varieties, smooth bundling, and tempting flavors in tobacco items explicitly intended for the adolescent market further epitomizes the business' shrewdness approach. Items like enhanced stogies and cigarillos, frequently with candy-like bundling, have attracted more youthful buyers, making another age of tobacco clients who might know nothing about the drawn out wellbeing results.

The idea of corporate social obligation (CSR) has additionally been controlled by the tobacco business as a component of its promoting procedure. All the while assuming a pretense of being socially capable, tobacco organizations have taken part in sponsorships of far-reaching developments, sports, and instructive projects. By falling in line with positive drives, the business tries to make a considerate picture, redirecting consideration from the damage brought about by their items.

The double-dealing of emotional wellness weaknesses is one more disturbing feature of the tobacco business' promoting strategies. Cigarettes, frequently promoted as a pressure reliever or a method for adapting to uneasiness, tap into the profound weaknesses of people battling with emotional wellness issues. The business profits by the longing for help and unwinding, making a misleading story that smoking can be an answer for emotional wellness challenges.

As of late, the ascent of elective nicotine conveyance frameworks, like e-cigarettes, has introduced another wilderness for the business to take advantage of. The smooth plan, subtle nature, and a heap of engaging flavors have made e-cigarettes alluring to a wide crowd, with a specific spotlight on baiting in youthful clients. The business' focusing of weak populaces stretches out to the advancement of these items as a popular and present day option in contrast to conventional cigarettes, in spite of worries about the obscure wellbeing impacts of vaping.

The adolescent vaping pestilence that followed uncovered the genuine degree of the business' ruthless practices. Organizations like Juul, which acquired reputation for their minimal, USB-like gadgets and captivating flavors, confronted allegations of purposefully advertising to youngsters. The flood in vaping among young people prompted far and wide wellbeing concerns and administrative examination, provoking a reconsideration of the business' showcasing strategies.

Past public lines, the tobacco business has decisively designated weak populaces in emerging nations. These areas, frequently missing strong tobacco control measures, became ripe justification for the business' extension. Forceful promoting strategies, joined with remiss guidelines, worked with the business' endeavors to lay out a traction in these business sectors.

The World Wellbeing Association's Structure Show on Tobacco Control (FCTC) expected to address the global components of tobacco control. Notwithstanding, the tobacco business effectively went against and campaigned against the FCTC, trying to subvert its arrangements and keep up with its impact in emerging nations. This resistance featured the business' readiness to take advantage of weak populaces internationally, putting benefit in front of general wellbeing on an overall scale.

The tobacco business' strategies of focusing on weak populaces reach out to its obstruction in open approach and political cycles. Through broad campaigning endeavors, crusade commitments, and partnerships with political figures, the business has affected regulation and administrative structures in support of its. The spinning entryway between the tobacco business and government organizations has raised worries about irreconcilable circumstances, compromising general wellbeing drives and focusing on the business' advantages over the prosperity of the populace.

One glaring illustration of this impact is the business' resistance to expanded tax collection on tobacco items. Higher assessments have been demonstrated to be a compelling apparatus in diminishing tobacco utilization, particularly among weak populaces with restricted discretionary cashflow. In any case, the tobacco business, driven by benefit thought processes, has reliably battled against charge increments, utilizing a scope of strategies to influence policymakers and forestall the execution of measures that could safeguard weak populaces.

The job of race and financial status in the tobacco business' promoting procedures can't be disregarded. Studies have shown that specific networks, especially those with lower financial status and higher extents of minority populaces, are excessively focused on by tobacco publicizing. The conscious arrangement of notices in these networks, combined with cost advancements and the accessibility of less expensive tobacco items, adds to wellbeing variations among various racial and financial gatherings.

Enhanced tobacco items, with their enticement for more youthful clients, have been especially pervasive in minority networks. The business' focusing of these networks mirrors an upsetting example of double-dealing, exploiting existing imbalances to additional its own advantages.

Despite mounting proof and public mindfulness, the tobacco business keeps on adjusting its methodologies to keep up with its hold on weak populaces. The utilization of web-based entertainment as a strong showcasing device has permitted the business to contact a worldwide crowd, impacting insights and conduct on an exceptional scale.

Online stages, with their capacity to target explicit socioeconomics, have become milestones for the business' advertising efforts, further intensifying the requirement for complete and refreshed administrative measures.

Endeavors to counter the tobacco business' double-dealing of weak populaces require a multi-pronged methodology. Fortifying and implementing guidelines to limit promoting, especially in places open to youth, is a vital stage. Executing and increasing government rates on tobacco items can assist with lessening openness, particularly in networks with restricted assets. General wellbeing efforts pointed toward dispersing the fantasies proliferated by the business and instructing weak populaces about the dangers of tobacco use are fundamental parts of an exhaustive technique.

Tending to the impact of the tobacco business in governmental issues requests more prominent straightforwardness and responsibility. Stricter guidelines on political commitments and campaigning exercises can assist with moderating the business' effect on open approach. Also, endeavors to diminish the business' contribution in general wellbeing direction, like stricter irreconcilable circumstance rules, are important to guarantee that the prosperity of the populace outweighs corporate interests.

The battle against the tobacco business' ruthless showcasing strategies likewise requires coordinated effort on a worldwide scale. Fortifying peaceful accords, like the FCTC, and advancing collaboration between nations can assist with making a unified front against the business' worldwide impact. By sharing prescribed procedures and illustrations learned, countries can by and large make progress toward safeguarding weak populaces and progressing worldwide general wellbeing.

All in all, the report on promoting systems focusing on weak populaces uncovers a disturbing story of double-dealing, control, and corporate ravenousness. The tobacco business, specifically, has consummated the craft of going after weak gatherings, from ladies and youngsters to networks with lower financial status. The business' strategies reach out past public lines, representing a worldwide danger to general wellbeing and requiring a planned and careful reaction.

To counter these deceptive practices, there should be a pledge to vigorous and versatile guidelines, public mindfulness missions, and global joint effort. Just through an exhaustive and supported exertion might we at any point desire to divulge the genuine degree of the tobacco business' double-dealing and safeguard weak populaces from the savage practices that focus on benefit over the wellbeing and prosperity of people and networks.

### 4.3 Legal battles and controversies surrounding the tobacco industry

The tobacco business has been enmeshed in a snare of fights in court and contentions that have molded its direction and the scene of general wellbeing. From the early claims that tried to consider the business responsible for the wellbeing results of smoking to later fights over promoting rehearses and arising items like e-cigarettes, the lawful field has been a landmark where the interests of general wellbeing and the tobacco business impact.

One of the earliest and most important fights in court against the tobacco business happened in the last 50% of the twentieth 100 years. As logical proof connecting smoking to cellular breakdown in the lungs and different sicknesses started to arise, people who had endured wellbeing side-effects because of smoking looked for lawful plan of action. These early cases made ready for an influx of suit that would on a very basic level test the business' practices.

The defining moment came during the 1950s and 1960s when milestone concentrates by scientists like Richard Doll and A. Bradford Slope laid out an unmistakable connection among smoking and cellular breakdown in the lungs. The Top health spokesperson's report in 1964 further cemented the logical agreement on the risks of smoking. Outfitted with this information, people and their legitimate delegates started claims against tobacco organizations, asserting that they had been hurt by the business' dishonest practices.

The legitimate scene moved emphatically with the expansion of legal claims. These claims, welcomed for the benefit of gatherings of people who had experienced comparative mischief, represented a huge danger to the tobacco business. Nonetheless, the business retaliated vivaciously, utilizing a scope of lawful strategies to challenge the legitimacy of the cases and postpone procedures.

The mind boggling and extended nature of these fights in court was exemplified by the situation of Cipollone v. Liggett Gathering, Inc. during the 1980s. Rose Cipollone's family documented a claim against Liggett Gathering, charging that the organization's cigarettes caused her cellular breakdown in the lungs and possible demise. The case dug into the complexities of caution names, promoting, and the business' information on wellbeing chances. While the jury at first granted harms to the Cipollone family, the choice was subsequently upset on request.

In spite of legitimate misfortunes, individual claims started to get momentum, and the combined load of these cases caused to notice the business' culpability. In 1998, the significant tobacco organizations arrived at a memorable settlement with 46 U.S. states, known as the Expert Settlement Understanding (MSA). The settlement expected tobacco organizations to pay billions of dollars yearly to the states, remunerating them for the medical services costs related with smoking-related diseases. It additionally forced limitations on promoting works on, precluding specific types of publicizing and sponsorship of social and games.

While the MSA denoted a critical triumph for general wellbeing backers and state legislatures, the fights in court were not even close to finished. The business confronted a surge of individual claims, including those brought by smokers experiencing smoking-related ailments. Immersed in an ocean of suit, significant tobacco organizations wound up at the focal point of a lawful bedlam that uncovered inward records uncovering a conscious system to make light of the habit-forming nature of nicotine and stifle data about the wellbeing dangers of smoking.

The business' inside reports, which became known during the revelation cycle in different claims, portrayed trickery and control. The reports showed that tobacco organizations knew about the wellbeing chances related with smoking, including the habit-forming properties of nicotine, yet effectively attempted to hide this data. This disclosure energized public shock and further fortified the lawful bodies of evidence against the business.

One essential second in this legitimate adventure was the declaration of seven tobacco industry Presidents before the US Congress in 1994. Having sworn to tell the truth, these chiefs conceded that nicotine was habit-forming and that smoking caused different illnesses, including cellular breakdown in the lungs. The broadcast hearings denoted a turning point, breaking the business' veneer of disavowal and uncovering its insight into the mischief brought about by its items.

The fights in court stretched out to issues of item risk and promoting rehearses. Tobacco organizations confronted allegations that they had controlled nicotine levels to improve dependence, designated weak populaces, and participated in misleading and tricky publicizing. These charges prodded an influx of individual and legal claims looking for remuneration for wellbeing harms, smoking-related sicknesses, and financial misfortunes.

The business' lawful difficulties were not bound to the US. In Canada, a weighty case unfurled during the 1990s known as the "Tobacco Wars." Territories in Canada looked to recuperate medical services costs related with smoking-related diseases from tobacco organizations. The case brought about a milestone settlement in 2008, where three significant tobacco organizations consented to pay billions of dollars to the regions more than a 25-year time frame.

As the fights in court unfurled, so did disclosures about the business' endeavors to sabotage general wellbeing arrangements and impact government direction. Interior reports uncovered the degree of the business' political impact, with campaigning endeavors, crusade commitments, and vital coalitions with political figures intended to shape regulation and administrative systems in support of its.

The spinning entryway between the tobacco business and government organizations raised worries about irreconcilable situations. Previous industry chiefs tracked down positions inside administrative bodies, making a view of compromised independent direction and ruining endeavors to carry out successful tobacco control measures.

This crossing point of industry and government further energized legitimate and moral discussions encompassing the guideline of an item with such significant wellbeing suggestions.

Global elements of the fights in court became obvious too. The World Wellbeing Association's Structure Show on Tobacco Control (FCTC), embraced in 2003, addressed a worldwide work to address the difficulties presented by the tobacco business. The FCTC tried to lay out worldwide norms for tobacco control, covering regions like publicizing, tax assessment, and bundling. Notwithstanding, the tobacco business effectively went against the FCTC, campaigning against its reception and trying to debilitate its arrangements.

Case and lawful difficulties connected with tobacco publicizing and bundling arose as basic landmarks. State run administrations all over the planet tried to execute realistic advance notice marks on cigarette bundles to convey the wellbeing dangers of smoking all the more actually. The tobacco business answered with lawful difficulties, contending that such measures encroached on its more right than wrong to business free discourse. This prompted a progression of fights in court, for certain nations effectively carrying out realistic advance notice marks in spite of the business' resistance.

The legitimate scene advanced with the rise of new items like e-cigarettes. The promoting and guideline of these items turned into a hostile issue, with the business situating them as a less unsafe option in contrast to conventional cigarettes. In any case, worries about the wellbeing impacts of vaping, particularly among youngsters, prompted lawful difficulties and administrative activities.

The young vaping pestilence, powered by the prominence of items like Juul, incited examinations and claims against e-cigarette makers. Allegations of tricky showcasing works on, focusing of underage clients, and minimizing wellbeing chances became central places of legitimate activity. The business confronted expanded investigation from controllers, legislators, and the general population, with calls for stricter guidelines on e-cigarettes and a reconsideration of their part in general wellbeing.

Fights in court likewise stretched out to the domain of protected innovation and global economic alliance. Tobacco organizations, confronting limitations on bundling and promoting in certain nations, depended on legitimate difficulties in view of economic alliance and protected innovation freedoms. These difficulties brought up complex issues about the harmony between general wellbeing goals and the assurance of business interests.

Endeavors to counter the tobacco business' legitimate moves and safeguard general wellbeing require continuous cautiousness and flexibility. Reinforcing and implementing tobacco control guidelines, especially in regions like promoting, bundling, and item revelations, stay vital. Strong legitimate systems that endure industry challenges and developing items are fundamental to exploring the intricate territory of tobacco guideline.

The job of promotion gatherings and general wellbeing associations in starting lawful activity couldn't possibly be more significant. These gatherings assume a urgent part in considering the business responsible, focusing on tricky practices, and upholding for strategies that focus on general wellbeing over corporate interests. The co-operation between legitimate specialists, scientists, and supporters turns into a strong power in standing up to the lawful difficulties presented by the tobacco business.

Worldwide participation is similarly essential, given the worldwide idea of the tobacco business. Reinforcing and extending the range of peaceful accords like the FCTC can assist with making a brought together front against industry obstruction and advance steady principles for tobacco control around the world. Lawful activities at the worldwide level can start trends and add to a worldwide system that safeguards general wellbeing from the business' strategies.

# Chapter 5

### The Health Toll

The contemporary world is set apart by its persistent speed, mind boggling interconnectedness, and the ceaseless quest for progress. In the midst of the transcending accomplishments of science, innovation, and civilization, a quiet cost frequently slips through the cracks — the cost for human wellbeing. This diverse test envelops actual prosperity as well as mental and social aspects, entwining with the texture of our regular routines in manners that are both unobtrusive and significant.

In the domain of actual wellbeing, the cost is obvious in the rising predominance of constant sicknesses. Current ways of life, described by stationary propensities, unfortunate dietary decisions, and the ubiquity of stress, add to a developing scourge of conditions like stoutness, diabetes, and cardiovascular infections. The human body, superbly versatile for what it's worth, battles to adapt to the extreme changes forced by the contemporary climate. As we drench ourselves in the advanced age, the alluring sparkle of screens spellbinds our consideration, frequently to the detriment of outside exercises and actual activity. The outcome is a general public that is progressively fastened to work areas and screens, forfeiting the regular rhythms of development that have molded human advancement for centuries.

Nourishment, a foundation of actual wellbeing, bears the heaviness of the cost too. The wealth of handled food varieties, weighed down with sugars, fats, and fake added substances, represents an imposing test to the body's sensitive balance. The ascent of cheap food culture, driven by accommodation and moderateness, further dissolves the nourishing groundwork of our weight control plans. Thus, we wind up in the confusing circumstance of having remarkable admittance to food, yet wrestling with ailing health in its different structures. The cost for actual wellbeing, typified by the growing waistlines of populaces around the world, is a powerful sign of the complicated transaction between human decisions and the climate that shapes them.

While actual wellbeing is a substantial indication of the cost, the elements of emotional well-being are similarly huge. The fast speed of current life, described by data over-burden and the unremitting requests of a hyperconnected world, demands a cost for the human brain. Stress, nervousness, and wretchedness have become unavoidable associates, penetrating the existences of people across assorted financial layers. The strain to succeed, combined with the consistent examination worked with by web-based entertainment, makes a favorable place for emotional well-being difficulties. The cost stretches out past the individual, penetrating families, working environments, and networks.

Innovation, a blade that cuts both ways in the contemporary story, assumes a focal part in forming the psychological wellness scene. On one hand, the computerized insurgency has democratized admittance to data, associating minds across mainlands and encouraging development. Then again, the relentless flood of warnings, the habit-forming charm of web-based entertainment, and the obscuring limits among work and individual life add to a psychological scene laden with difficulties. The cost for psychological well-being isn't restricted to the virtual domain; it reverberations in the blessed lobbies of instructive foundations, corporate workplaces, and the isolation of homes.

Social wellbeing, the frequently ignored element of prosperity, is entwined with the texture of human connections. The cost for social wellbeing is apparent in the disintegration of local area bonds, the fraying of family ties, and the unavoidable feeling of disengagement that hides underneath the outer layer of current cultures. Urbanization, the embodiment of progress in many regards, frequently cuts off the binds that tight spot people to their underlying foundations. The quest for individual objectives, driven by cultural assumptions and financial goals, can prompt an aggregate disregard of the social biological system that supports us.

The cost for social wellbeing stretches out to the domain of relational connections. The approach of online entertainment, while cultivating virtual associations, amazingly separates people from the wealth of up close and personal cooperations. The organized stories introduced on computerized stages make a contorted reality, energizing the perpetual human propensity to look at and contend. Bona fide associations, the bedrock of social wellbeing, frequently succumb to the shallow charm of online personas.

The cost for wellbeing, in its all encompassing sense, is exacerbated by ecological variables. The planet, troubled by the overabundances of human utilization and industrialization, reflects the cost as environmental change, contamination, and the exhaustion of normal assets. The air we inhale, the water we drink, and the food we polish off bear the engravings of natural debasement. The cost for human wellbeing, unpredictably connected to the strength of the planet, highlights the inseparable association between the prosperity of people and the biological systems they occupy.

The cost for wellbeing, in its horde structures, brings up principal issues about the direction of human advancement. Will a general public that forfeits the strength of its residents in the persevering quest for mechanical, monetary, and social progression genuinely be considered fruitful? The Catch 22s inborn in this question reverberation through the halls of time, testing the actual groundworks of the accounts that characterize human progress.

Tending to the cost for wellbeing requires a change in outlook — a reexamination of cultural needs, individual decisions, and the actual meaning of progress. The arrangements lie not just in that frame of mind of clinical mediations but rather in the more extensive areas of schooling, strategy, and social standards. It requests a recalibration of values, setting human prosperity at the very front of the aggregate plan.

In the domain of actual wellbeing, the way ahead includes a re-visitation of the basics of adjusted living. Training assumes a vital part in this cycle, enabling people with the information to pursue informed decisions about their ways of life. Drives that advance active work, admittance to nutritious food, and an all encompassing way to deal with prosperity can make ready for a better society. Strategy mediations, going from metropolitan arranging that focuses on green spaces to guidelines that control the abundances of the food business, are fundamental parts of the arrangement.

The cost for psychological well-being requires a nuanced approach that recognizes the intricacies of the cutting edge mind. Instructive educational programs that focus on capacity to appreciate people on a profound level, versatility, and strategies for dealing with stress can prepare people to explore the difficulties of the computerized age. Working environment strategies that focus on balance between serious and fun activities, emotional well-being days, and strong conditions cultivate a culture of prosperity. Destigmatizing emotional well-being issues, advancing open exchange, and upgrading admittance to emotional well-being administrations are basic strides towards building a general public that esteems the psychological prosperity of its residents.

Social wellbeing, frequently consigned to the fringe of public talk, requests a reviving of local area bonds and the development of significant connections. Drives that cultivate local area commitment, commend variety, and address the main drivers of social disengagement can add to a dynamic social texture.

Approaches that focus on family support, parental leave, and adaptable work plans perceive the reliance of individual and cultural prosperity. Past the advanced facade of virtual entertainment, valid human associations, grounded in sympathy and understanding, are the antitoxin to the cost for social wellbeing.

The cost for wellbeing, interlaced with ecological corruption, highlights the basic of maintainable living. Strategies that focus on natural protection, sustainable power, and eco-accommodating practices contribute not exclusively to the strength of the planet yet additionally to the wellbeing of its occupants. Individual decisions, from manageable utilization examples to eco-cognizant ways of life, structure the bedrock of a harmonious connection among humankind and the climate. The acknowledgment that the soundness of people and the strength of the planet are indistinguishable is a basic step towards a future that focuses on the prosperity of every living being.

At its center, tending to the cost for wellbeing requires an aggregate change in cognizance — an acknowledgment that genuine advancement is estimated in financial files and mechanical progressions as well as in the wellbeing and bliss of people. It requires a rethinking of cultural standards, values, and desires, rising above the restricted limits of transient increases and individual pursuits. The cost for wellbeing, completely, is a source of inspiration — a call to manufacture a future where the quest for progress blends with the safeguarding of human, mental, and social prosperity.

All in all, the cost for wellbeing is a diverse test that pervades the actual texture of contemporary presence. From the actual elements of ongoing sicknesses to the perplexing scene of mental and social prosperity, the cost appears in bunch structures. Innovation, while a guide of progress, raises serious questions about emotional wellbeing, and the quest for individual achievement frequently comes to the detriment of social associations. Ecological debasement, a frequently neglected aspect, reflects the cost for human wellbeing, building up the interconnectedness of all life on The planet.

Tending to the cost for wellbeing requires an all encompassing methodology that rises above the limits of conventional storehouses. It requests a recalibration of cultural qualities, individual decisions, and the actual meaning of progress. The arrangements lie in the domain of clinical mediations as well as in the more extensive spaces of training, strategy, and social standards. A future that focuses on the prosperity of people is definitely not an idealistic dream however a substantial chance — one that requires aggregate activity, cognizant decisions, and a promise to fashioning a way where progress and wellbeing coincide as one.

### 5.1 In-depth exploration of smoking-related health issues

The unavoidable demonstration of smoking, notwithstanding many years of general wellbeing efforts and broad logical examination, keeps on being a critical worldwide wellbeing concern. The perplexing snare of smoking-related medical problems traverses a range that envelops not just the deeply grounded dangers of cellular breakdown in the lungs and respiratory sicknesses yet in addition a heap of other medical issue influencing practically every organ framework in the human body. This inside and out investigation expects to take apart the multi-layered effect of smoking, revealing insight into the physiological, mental, and cultural elements of this unavoidable propensity.

At the front of smoking-related medical problems is the factual relationship with respiratory infections. Inward breath of tobacco smoke, a complicated combination of thousands of synthetic compounds, straightforwardly attacks the fragile designs of the lungs. Persistent obstructive pneumonic sickness (COPD), including conditions like constant bronchitis and emphysema, remains as an obvious demonstration of the horrendous impacts of smoking on respiratory wellbeing. The inward breath of aggravations and poisons triggers irritation, compromises aviation route capability, and prompts the ever-evolving weakening of lung tissue.

Cellular breakdown in the lungs, maybe the most famous result of smoking, is unpredictably connected to the cancer-causing agents present in tobacco smoke. The change of typical lung cells into threatening partners is an intricate exchange of hereditary transformations and natural openings. The stunning pervasiveness of cellular breakdown in the lungs among smokers fills in as a grave sign of the preventable idea of this sickness. The effect reaches out past the person, with handed-down cigarette smoke openness representing a huge gamble to non-smokers, particularly in restricted spaces like homes and working environments.

While the respiratory framework endures the worst part of smoking-related medical problems, the cardiovascular framework isn't saved. Smoking is a significant gamble factor for cardiovascular illnesses, including coronary supply route infection, stroke, and fringe vascular sickness. The vasoconstrictive impacts of nicotine, combined with the supportive of fiery and favorable to thrombotic properties of other tobacco parts, make a milieu helpful for the improvement of atherosclerosis — the fundamental cycle behind numerous cardiovascular circumstances. The outcomes are critical, with smokers confronting a raised gamble of cardiovascular failures, strokes, and vascular entanglements that contribute fundamentally to worldwide horribleness and mortality.

Past the domain of actual wellbeing, smoking demands a cost for mental prosperity. The multifaceted connection among smoking and psychological wellness problems, especially melancholy and uneasiness, is a subject of developing interest and concern.

While people frequently go to smoking as a way of dealing with especially difficult times for pressure or profound trouble, the habit-forming nature of nicotine intensifies the intricacy of the relationship. The impermanent help presented by smoking is a blade that cuts both ways, as it propagates a pattern of reliance that extends the weaving of smoking with emotional wellness challenges.

The effect of smoking on conceptive wellbeing is a frequently ignored aspect. Both male and female fruitfulness are unfavorably impacted by smoking, with suggestions for origination and pregnancy results. In guys, smoking is related with diminished sperm quality, changed sperm motility, and an expanded gamble of erectile brokenness. In females, smoking adds to ripeness issues, complexities during pregnancy, and unfavorable results for the creating embryo. The transgenerational impacts of smoking highlight the broad results that stretch out past the singular smoker to affect people in the future.

The cost for oral wellbeing is one more aspect of smoking-related medical problems that warrants consideration. Smoking is a significant gamble factor for periodontal illnesses, which influence the supporting designs of the teeth. The vasoconstrictive and immunosuppressive impacts of smoking trade off the body's capacity to battle contaminations, prompting the expansion of microorganisms in the oral pit. The outcome is a fountain of fiery cycles that add to gum sickness, tooth misfortune, and in general oral wellbeing crumbling. Moreover, smoking is a huge gamble factor for oral malignant growths, further stressing the malicious consequences for the whole oral cavity.

Smoking-related medical problems stretch out past individual wellbeing to incorporate more extensive cultural ramifications. The monetary weight of smoking-related sicknesses is faltering, with direct medical care costs, efficiency misfortunes, and the burden on medical care frameworks forcing an imposing test. The far reaching influences of smoking touch each side of society, from families wrestling with the results of a friend or family member's smoking-related disease to networks troubled by the aggregate effect on general wellbeing.

Endeavors to address smoking-related medical problems have been complex, going from administrative measures to general wellbeing efforts. The execution of tobacco control strategies, including tax collection, promoting limitations, and without smoke conditions, plays had a critical impact in checking smoking rates in certain districts. General wellbeing efforts, intended to bring issues to light about the risks of smoking and advance smoking suspension, have additionally added to moving cultural perspectives towards this inescapable propensity.

Smoking end, the foundation of preventive endeavors, is a complicated and testing venture for some people. Nicotine compulsion, combined with the mental and social parts of smoking, makes an imposing obstruction to stopping.

Smoking suspension mediations include a range of approaches, from pharmacological guides, for example, nicotine substitution treatment to conduct intercessions and backing programs. The acknowledgment of smoking as a persistent backsliding condition highlights the significance of custom fitted and extensive procedures to help people on their way to stopping.

The worldwide scene of smoking-related medical problems is set apart by huge abberations. While smoking rates have declined in some big league salary nations, they keep on ascending in low-and center pay countries, frequently determined by designated promoting techniques of tobacco organizations. The weight of smoking-related sicknesses lopsidedly influences weak populaces, intensifying existing wellbeing disparities. Endeavors to address smoking-related medical problems must, consequently, consider the social determinants of wellbeing, recognizing the diversity that shapes examples of tobacco use and its ramifications.

Arising patterns, like the ascent of electronic cigarettes (e-cigarettes), add a layer of intricacy to the scene of smoking-related medical problems. While defenders contend that e-cigarettes offer a less hurtful option in contrast to conventional smoking, concerns continue with respect to their drawn out wellbeing and the possibility to act as a door to customary smoking, particularly among youth. The unique idea of the tobacco scene highlights the continuous requirement for examination, reconnaissance, and versatile general wellbeing systems to address advancing examples of tobacco use.

All in all, the investigation of smoking-related medical problems uncovers an embroidery of difficulties that reach out a long ways past the limits of respiratory sicknesses. From the cardiovascular framework to emotional wellness, conceptive wellbeing, oral wellbeing, and cultural ramifications, smoking creates a long shaded area over individual and aggregate prosperity. The excursion towards a smoke-liberated world requires a thorough and deliberate exertion, enveloping strategy measures, general wellbeing mediations, and a cultural change in perspectives towards smoking. As we disentangle the layers of smoking-related medical problems, the basic to shield current and people in the future from the preventable damages of tobacco use turns out to be progressively obvious — a source of inspiration that reverberates in the hallways of general wellbeing as well as in the actual pith of human prosperity.

**5.2 Personal testimonies of individuals affected by smoking-related diseases**

The effect of smoking-related sicknesses resounds a long ways past clinical measurements and epidemiological patterns. Behind the numbers lie profoundly private accounts of people whose lives have been irreversibly adjusted by the outcomes of tobacco use. These individual declarations act as impactful tokens of the human cost claimed by smoking, revealing insight into the physical, profound, and social components of the excursion through sickness.

One ongoing idea that ties these declarations is the guileful idea of dependence. Numerous people share a story of blamelessness lost, describing the underlying charm of smoking and the continuous plummet into reliance. The underlying puff, frequently taken during youthfulness or youthful adulthood, is depicted as an apparently innocuous demonstration — a transitional experience or a statement of defiance. Little do these people expect the strong hold that nicotine will come to apply on their lives.

As habit grabs hold, the declarations frequently mirror a mind boggling interaction of variables adding to the propagation of smoking. Stress, social impacts, and the ceremonial idea of smoking become laced with the physiological desires, making a considerable obstruction to stopping. The battle to break liberated from the grasp of compulsion turns into a characterizing part in these stories, set apart by a progression of endeavors and backslides, each joined by a restored feeling of assurance and disappointment.

The actual cost of smoking, clearly depicted in these declarations, appears in a heap of ways. Respiratory side effects, like constant hack, windedness, and wheezing, become unwanted buddies in the regular routines of people wrestling with smoking-related illnesses. The steady movement from minor inconvenience to incapacitating side effects is a typical subject, with many communicating a feeling of treachery by their own bodies.

For those determined to have ongoing obstructive pneumonic infection (COPD), the stories frequently dive into the difficulties of living with a condition that tenaciously decreases respiratory capability. The basic demonstration of breathing, once underestimated, turns into a relentless undertaking, joined by the steady consciousness of the restricted limit of one's lungs. Intensifications, set apart by episodes of expanded side effects and uplifted trouble, accentuate the all around exhausting excursion of people living with COPD.

The phantom of cellular breakdown in the lungs creates an especially serious shaded area in these declarations. The conclusion is often depicted as a life changing second, denoting a distinct takeoff from the direction imagined by those impacted. The stories enlighten the close to home choppiness that goes with the acknowledgment of mortality and the overwhelming possibility of standing up to an imposing foe inside one's own body.

The cost for emotional well-being is a repetitive topic in these declarations, highlighting the multifaceted connection among smoking and mental prosperity. The shame related with smoking-related illnesses adds an extra layer of intricacy, with people wrestling with the actual difficulties as well as with cultural discernments and self-fault. Wretchedness and uneasiness, frequently exacerbated by the disconnecting idea of constant sickness, become imposing enemies in the fight for generally prosperity.

The effect on connections is one more aspect investigated in these individual declarations. The stress on familial bonds is unmistakable, with companions, youngsters, and more distant family individuals frequently filling in as the two mainstays of help and observers to the steady downfall of wellbeing. The responsibility and distress communicated by people who feel they have troubled their friends and family with the results of their smoking add a strong layer to these stories.

Parental declarations, specifically, offer an exceptional point of view on the intergenerational effect of smoking. The torment of guardians who should stand up to the truth of their smoking impacting the soundness of their kids is an intermittent subject. From the pain of pregnant moms wrestling with the apprehension about unfriendly results to the responsibility experienced by guardians whose youngsters foster respiratory issues because of handed-down cigarette smoke openness, these declarations feature the extensive outcomes of smoking on the nuclear family.

The monetary strain related with smoking-related illnesses arises as a consistent idea, with people describing the oppressive expenses of clinical consideration, prescriptions, and, at times, the failure to work due to disintegrating wellbeing. The convergence of wellbeing and financial status becomes obvious, with impeded people confronting intensified difficulties in getting to satisfactory medical care and backing administrations.

Regardless of the unavoidable difficulties portrayed in these declarations, strength and the quest for trust radiate through. Numerous people share accounts of groundbreaking minutes that act as impetuses for change. Whether enlivened by the introduction of a grandkid, the distinct acknowledgment of mortality, or a urgent discussion with a medical services supplier, these minutes mark a defining moment in the excursion towards smoking end and by and large wellbeing improvement.

Smoking discontinuance endeavors highlight unmistakably in these declarations, with people describing the procedures utilized, the mishaps confronted, and the victories celebrated en route. The aggregate insight shared by the individuals who have effectively stopped fills in as a wellspring of motivation for others actually exploring the troublesome way towards freedom from nicotine compulsion.

The job of medical care experts in these stories is significant. The sympathy and direction given by specialists, attendants, and other medical care suppliers arise as helps for people wrestling with smoking-related sicknesses. The special interactions produced in the medical services setting frequently rise above the clinical domain, offering everyday reassurance and a feeling of organization in the excursion towards better wellbeing.

As these individual declarations unfurl, it becomes obvious that the excursion through smoking-related illnesses is certainly not a single one. Encouraging groups of people, both formal and casual, assume a urgent part in the stories of people impacted by smoking. From help gatherings and guiding administrations to the resolute consolation of loved ones, the shared part of the battle against smoking-related sicknesses is a common subject.

The craving to share these declarations is regularly determined by a feeling of backing — an intense expectation that the examples gained from individual encounters will impact others, deterring them from the way of tobacco use or empowering those generally on that way to look for help. The stories act as useful examples, encouraging society to go up against the unforgiving real factors of smoking and to focus on preventive estimates that can save people and their families from the desolates of tobacco-related diseases.

All in all, the individual declarations of people impacted by smoking-related sicknesses offer a piercing and complex point of view on the significant effect of tobacco use. These stories rise above clinical portrayals and factual examinations, digging into the profound, social, and mental elements of the excursion through ailment. From the tricky idea of dependence on the actual cost for respiratory and cardiovascular wellbeing, the stories illustrate the difficulties looked by those wrestling with smoking-related sicknesses.

These declarations likewise enlighten the crossing points among smoking and emotional wellness, connections, monetary prosperity, and cultural insights. The versatility and trust implanted in these stories act as signals of motivation for others confronting comparative difficulties, highlighting the groundbreaking force of individual organization and the help of medical services experts and networks.

As these individual declarations wind around together an embroidery of lived encounters, they entice society to face the unforgiving real factors of smoking and to focus on extensive systems for counteraction and smoking end. The source of inspiration isn't just an aggregate liability yet an empathetic reaction to the voices that reverberation through these accounts — an update that, behind each measurement, there is a remarkable and important story that should be heard, comprehended, and tended to with sympathy and criticalness.

### 5.3 Economic burden on healthcare systems due to smoking-related illnesses

The financial weight forced on medical services frameworks by smoking-related diseases is an imposing test that reverberates worldwide. Past the singular affliction and misfortune, the monetary stress on medical services foundations is significant, affecting financial plans, assets, and the general maintainability of medical services frameworks. This investigation dives into the complex components of the financial weight related with smoking-related diseases, revealing insight into the immediate and aberrant costs that resound through medical services frameworks.

At the center of the monetary test lies the immediate medical services costs brought about in the determination, therapy, and the executives of smoking-related ailments.

The range of illnesses credited to smoking — going from respiratory circumstances like persistent obstructive pneumonic sickness (COPD) to cardiovascular infections and different malignant growths — requests broad clinical consideration. Hospitalizations, demonstrative methods, drugs, and medical procedures comprise huge parts of these immediate expenses.

The weight on medical services frameworks is most clear with regards to cellular breakdown in the lungs, a sickness unequivocally connected to tobacco use. The complex and asset escalated nature of malignant growth care, including a medical procedure, chemotherapy, radiation treatment, and steady intercessions, overburdens medical care financial plans. The financial ramifications stretch out to the administration of cutting edge phases of cellular breakdown in the lungs, where palliative consideration and end-of-life mediations add to the general expense.

Persistent sicknesses like COPD, frequently an outcome of long haul smoking, require progressing clinical consideration and mediations. The intensifications and complexities related with COPD lead to repetitive hospitalizations and trauma center visits, adding to the financial cost. The interest for respiratory meds, oxygen treatment, and restoration benefits further builds the immediate medical services costs related with smoking-related respiratory diseases.

Cardiovascular sicknesses, one more significant classification of smoking-related diseases, contribute altogether to the monetary weight on medical services frameworks. The administration of conditions like coronary corridor illness, stroke, and fringe vascular infection includes a range of intercessions, including drugs, interventional techniques, and careful mediations. The drawn out care expected to address the constant idea of cardiovascular sicknesses enhances the monetary stress on medical services assets.

The financial effect isn't restricted to the treatment stage; preventive measures, screening projects, and general wellbeing efforts pointed toward moderating the pervasiveness of smoking-related diseases additionally order significant assets. Against smoking drives, for example, smoking suspension programs and instructive missions, require financing for advancement, execution, and effort endeavors. The designation of assets to preventive techniques addresses an interest in turning away future medical care costs, highlighting the monetary reasoning for proactive general wellbeing measures.

The aberrant expenses related with smoking-related sicknesses add one more layer to the financial weight on medical care frameworks. Efficiency misfortunes because of truancy, handicap, and untimely mortality comprise a huge part of these backhanded expenses. People wrestling with smoking-related ailments frequently face difficulties in keeping up with standard work, prompting pay misfortune and expanded reliance on friendly emotionally supportive networks.

The effect on efficiency is especially articulated with regards to persistent respiratory circumstances like COPD. Shortness of breath, weakness, and the roundabout idea of intensifications every now and again bring about constraints in work limit. The total impact is a labor force that isn't just troubled by the immediate expenses of medical services yet in addition by the roundabout expenses originating from reduced efficiency and the related financial consequences for the two people and society.

The financial results reach out to the nuclear family, with parental figures frequently enduring the worst part of the providing care liabilities. The time and exertion put by relatives in offering help to people with smoking-related diseases bring about efficiency misfortunes that stretch out past the impacted person to the more extensive local area. The open door cost of providing care, with regards to inevitable business and monetary commitments, adds to the by and large financial weight on society.

The drawn out incapacity related with smoking-related diseases, especially those influencing the respiratory and cardiovascular frameworks, overwhelms handicap support programs. Incapacity benefits, restoration administrations, and social help programs cause costs that are intelligent of the persistent and frequently moderate nature of smoking-related sicknesses. The financial repercussions stretch out to protection frameworks, with expanded claims and payouts connected with handicap and life coverage for people impacted by smoking-related ailments.

The monetary weight on medical services frameworks is additionally exacerbated by the increased usage of medical services assets by people with smoking-related ailments. Trauma center visits, hospitalizations, and particular consideration add to the general stress on medical services framework. The interest for symptomatic methodology, imaging review, and lab tests adds to the expense of medical care conveyance, as does the requirement for continuous checking and the board of constant circumstances.

The worldwide size of the financial weight is clear with regards to medical care variations. Weak populaces, frequently with restricted admittance to preventive administrations and medical care assets, bear a lopsided portion of the financial outcomes related with smoking-related diseases. Variations in medical services access and results enhance the financial weight on medical services frameworks, as deferred or lacking consideration prompts more extreme sickness appearances and expanded medical care use.

The financial test isn't static; it develops over the long run as the commonness of smoking-related diseases varies and medical care costs keep on rising. Maturing populaces, with their expanded weakness to ongoing infections, represent extra difficulties to medical services frameworks. The requirement for creative and practical mediations becomes basic even with these segment shifts and the related ascent in the commonness of smoking-related sicknesses.

The financial weight on medical care frameworks meets with more extensive general wellbeing challenges, making a complicated snare of interrelated issues. The burden on medical care financial plans restricts the assets accessible for other fundamental wellbeing administrations, adding to a fountain impact that compromises in general medical services quality. The opposition for restricted assets requires hard choices in regards to asset designation, with possible consequences for the evenhanded appropriation of medical care administrations.

Tending to the financial weight of smoking-related diseases requires an exhaustive and incorporated approach that includes counteraction, treatment, and backing. Smoking suspension programs, with their capability to decrease the occurrence of smoking-related sicknesses, address a financially savvy interest in populace wellbeing. Complete tobacco control strategies, including tax assessment, promoting limitations, and sans smoke conditions, contribute not exclusively to lessening smoking rates yet additionally to relieving the monetary outcomes related with tobacco use.

Creative models of care, stressing preventive techniques and local area based mediations, hold guarantee in enhancing medical services asset usage. The coordination of telemedicine and computerized wellbeing advances can upgrade admittance to mind, particularly for people in remote or underserved regions. Cooperative endeavors between medical care frameworks, general wellbeing organizations, and local area associations can cultivate a synergistic way to deal with tending to the monetary weight of smoking-related diseases.

The monetary contention for putting resources into smoking end and preventive measures is built up by the potential for significant expense investment funds over the long haul. The decrease in medical services usage, efficiency misfortunes, and handicap related costs related with lower smoking rates add to a positive monetary effect. Financial displaying concentrates reliably show the good expense viability of smoking discontinuance mediations, giving a convincing reasoning to supported interest in tobacco control.

Worldwide cooperation is critical in tending to the worldwide financial weight of smoking-related sicknesses. Shared systems, examples learned, and cooperative exploration endeavors add to an aggregate methodology that rises above public limits. Associations like the World Wellbeing Association (WHO) assume a urgent part in organizing worldwide endeavors to battle tobacco use, underscoring the interconnectedness of wellbeing challenges and the requirement for a bound together reaction.

All in all, the monetary weight on medical services frameworks because of smoking-related sicknesses is a complicated and diverse test with sweeping results. The immediate medical services costs caused in the conclusion and therapy of smoking-related sicknesses, combined with the backhanded expenses originating from efficiency misfortunes and handicap, make a significant burden on medical care spending plans.

The financial test converges with more extensive general medical problems, accentuating the requirement for thorough techniques that include avoidance, therapy, and backing.

Interests in smoking end programs, tobacco control arrangements, and imaginative models of care address moral objectives as well as sound financial choices. The potential for significant expense investment funds over the long haul, combined with the positive effect on populace wellbeing, highlights the significance of supported endeavors to address.

The financial weight on medical services frameworks because of smoking-related sicknesses is an imposing and complex test that has significant ramifications for general wellbeing, monetary obligation, and the general prosperity of social orders across the globe. As we explore the complexities of this issue, it becomes apparent that the effect stretches out a long ways past the singular smoker, influencing medical care foundation, asset designation, and the actual texture of medical care frameworks.

At the core of the monetary test lies the immediate medical care costs related with the finding, therapy, and the executives of smoking-related ailments. These circumstances, going from respiratory illnesses like constant obstructive aspiratory sickness (COPD) to cardiovascular infections and different malignant growths, request broad clinical consideration. Hospitalizations, demonstrative methodology, drugs, and careful mediations comprise significant parts of these immediate expenses, overburdening medical services financial plans.

Cellular breakdown in the lungs, unequivocally connected to tobacco use, stands apart as a great representation of the monetary weight on medical care frameworks. The complex idea of disease care, including a medical procedure, chemotherapy, radiation treatment, and strong intercessions, adds to the by and large financial cost. The monetary ramifications reach out to the administration of cutting edge phases of cellular breakdown in the lungs, where palliative consideration and end-of-life mediations further raise the immediate medical services costs.

Constant infections like COPD, frequently a result of long haul smoking, require progressing clinical consideration and intercessions. Intensifications and difficulties related with COPD lead to intermittent hospitalizations and trauma center visits, adding to the monetary weight. The interest for respiratory meds, oxygen treatment, and recovery benefits further builds the immediate medical services costs related with smoking-related respiratory sicknesses.

Cardiovascular infections, one more significant classification of smoking-related sicknesses, fundamentally add to the monetary stress on medical services frameworks. The administration of conditions like coronary vein infection, stroke, and fringe vascular illness includes a range of intercessions, including prescriptions, interventional techniques, and careful mediations. The drawn out care expected to address the persistent idea of cardiovascular infections intensifies the monetary weight on medical services assets.

The monetary ramifications are not restricted to the treatment stage alone; preventive measures, screening projects, and general wellbeing efforts pointed toward relieving the predominance of smoking-related ailments likewise order critical assets. Hostile to smoking drives, including smoking end programs and instructive missions, require subsidizing for improvement, execution, and effort endeavors. The distribution of assets to preventive methodologies addresses an interest in deflecting future medical care costs, highlighting the financial reasoning for proactive general wellbeing measures.

Past the immediate medical care costs, the financial weight on medical care frameworks reaches out to aberrant costs that emerge from the results of smoking-related ailments. Efficiency misfortunes because of non-attendance, handicap, and untimely mortality structure a significant part of these backhanded expenses. People wrestling with smoking-related sicknesses frequently face difficulties in keeping up with ordinary business, prompting pay misfortune and expanded reliance on friendly emotionally supportive networks.

The effect on efficiency is especially articulated with regards to persistent respiratory circumstances like COPD. Side effects like windedness, weakness, and the roundabout idea of intensifications much of the time bring about constraints in work limit. The combined impact is a labor force troubled by the immediate expenses of medical services as well as by the roundabout expenses originating from lessened efficiency and the related monetary repercussions for the two people and society.

The financial outcomes stretch out to the nuclear family, where parental figures frequently endure the worst part of providing care liabilities. The time and exertion put by relatives in offering help to people with smoking-related diseases bring about efficiency misfortunes that reach out past the impacted person to the more extensive local area. The open door cost of providing care, regarding inevitable work and financial commitments, adds to the in general monetary weight on society.

Long haul handicap related with smoking-related diseases, especially those influencing the respiratory and cardiovascular frameworks, overburdens inability support programs. Incapacity benefits, restoration administrations, and social help programs cause costs intelligent of the ongoing and frequently moderate nature of smoking-related illnesses. The monetary implications stretch out to protection frameworks, with expanded claims and payouts connected with handicap and extra security for people impacted by smoking-related diseases.

The uplifted use of medical care assets by people with smoking-related ailments offers further to the monetary weight on medical services frameworks. Trauma center visits, hospitalizations, and specific consideration intensify the stress on medical care framework. The interest for indicative methods, imaging review, and research facility tests adds to the expense of medical services conveyance, as does the requirement for progressing observing and the board of persistent circumstances.

These monetary difficulties cross with more extensive general medical problems, making a complicated snare of interrelated concerns. Maturing populaces, with their expanded vulnerability to ongoing sicknesses, represent extra difficulties to medical services frameworks. The requirement for imaginative and financially savvy mediations becomes basic notwithstanding these segment shifts and the related ascent in the predominance of smoking-related sicknesses.

Tending to the financial weight of smoking-related sicknesses requires a thorough and coordinated approach that envelops counteraction, therapy, and backing. Smoking end programs, with their capability to lessen the occurrence of smoking-related sicknesses, address a practical interest in populace wellbeing. Extensive tobacco control approaches, including tax collection, publicizing limitations, and sans smoke conditions, contribute not exclusively to diminishing smoking rates yet additionally to relieving the financial outcomes related with tobacco use.

Creative models of care, stressing preventive methodologies and local area based mediations, hold guarantee in streamlining medical services asset use. The combination of telemedicine and advanced wellbeing innovations can upgrade admittance to mind, particularly for people in remote or underserved regions. Cooperative endeavors between medical care frameworks, general wellbeing offices, and local area associations can cultivate a synergistic way to deal with tending to the monetary weight of smoking-related sicknesses.

The monetary contention for putting resources into smoking discontinuance and preventive measures is supported by the potential for significant expense reserve funds over the long haul. The decrease in medical services usage, efficiency misfortunes, and handicap related costs related with lower smoking rates add to a positive financial effect. Monetary displaying concentrates reliably exhibit the ideal expense viability of smoking end mediations, giving a convincing reasoning to supported interest in tobacco control.

Worldwide cooperation is significant in tending to the worldwide financial weight of smoking-related diseases. Shared systems, examples learned, and cooperative exploration endeavors add to an aggregate methodology that rises above public limits. Associations like the World Wellbeing Association (WHO) assume a significant part in planning worldwide endeavors to battle tobacco use, underlining the interconnectedness of wellbeing challenges and the requirement for a bound together reaction.

All in all, the monetary weight on medical services frameworks because of smoking-related diseases is a perplexing and complex test with broad results. The immediate medical services costs related with the finding and therapy of smoking-related sicknesses, combined with the circuitous expenses originating from efficiency misfortunes and handicap, make a significant burden on medical care financial plans.

The financial test meets with more extensive general medical problems, accentuating the requirement for complete procedures that incorporate anticipation, therapy, and backing.

Interests in smoking end programs, tobacco control approaches, and imaginative models of care address moral goals as well as sound monetary choices. The potential for significant expense reserve funds over the long haul, combined with the positive effect on populace wellbeing, highlights the significance of supported endeavors to address the financial weight of smoking-related ailments. As medical services frameworks wrestle with the multifaceted difficulties presented by tobacco use, the basic to focus on preventive measures turns out to be progressively clear — a source of inspiration that reverberates in the hallways of medical services organizations as well as in the more extensive fields of strategy, general wellbeing, and worldwide coordinated effort.

# Chapter 6

### Breaking the Chains – Quitting Challenges

Breaking liberated from the chains that tight spot us is a widespread human goal. Whether these chains manifest as cultural assumptions, individual propensities, or mental hindrances, the excursion towards freedom is full of difficulties. Stopping, in its different structures, typifies the quintessence of this battle. It is a course of unraveling oneself from the natural, the agreeable, and at times, the horrendous.

The choice to break free frequently originates from an acknowledgment that the present status of undertakings is as of now not valid. It very well may be a task that smothers innovativeness, a relationship that has run its course, or an enslavement that has assumed command. Stopping, notwithstanding, is more difficult than one might expect. The very word conveys meanings of disappointment and shortcoming. Society frequently sees stopping as an acquiescence, an absence of tirelessness. However, is it generally so?

In truth, stopping can be a strong demonstration of self-protection and development. It requires one's very own profound comprehension needs, needs, and limits. The excursion to break liberated from chains is a groundbreaking cycle that requests mental fortitude, versatility, and a readiness to confront the unexplored world. This exposition investigates the different features of stopping difficulties, digging into the purposes for the choice to stop, the cultural insights encompassing it, and the self-awareness that frequently goes with such a striking decision.

At the core of stopping lies the acknowledgment of discontent. It's the affirmation that business as usual is at this point not satisfactory, that there exists a misalignment between one's real self and the ongoing conditions. This acknowledgment, be that as it may, is a two sided deal. On one hand, it makes the way for change and development; on the other, it compels one to defy awkward insights.

Take, for example, the expert circle. Numerous people secure themselves caught in positions that don't line up with their interests or values. The underlying fervor of a new position can wear off, abandoning a feeling of dreariness and disappointment. The choice to stop such a task isn't a confirmation of rout but instead an acknowledgment of the requirement for arrangement between private qualities and expert pursuits.

Likewise, connections can become chains that tight spot as opposed to bonds that feed. Whether it's a heartfelt organization, a kinship, or a familial tie, it is many times considered to be untouchable to stop a relationship. Society will in general esteem perseverance and unwaveringness, at times to the detriment of individual prosperity. Notwithstanding, perceiving when a relationship has become harmful or unfulfilling is a demonstration of confidence. Stopping, in this unique circumstance, turns into a gallant step towards a better close to home scene.

Addictions, maybe the most unmistakable chains, apply a strong hang on people. Substance misuse, habitual ways of behaving, and different types of compulsion can feel difficult. Stopping, in this unique circumstance, is a fight against oneself. Breaking liberated from the chains of enslavement needs outside help as well as an interior change. It requests a fair a showdown with one's weaknesses and a pledge to an alternate, better way.

The cultural impression of stopping is profoundly instilled. Since the beginning, people are shown the ideals of steadiness and tirelessness. While these characteristics are without a doubt significant, an unquestioning obligation to persevere notwithstanding difficulty can prompt an existence of calm distress. Society's accentuation on progress frequently eclipses the significance of satisfaction and individual prosperity.

The disgrace joined to stopping can be a considerable boundary. It's as though stopping is inseparable from surrendering, as though the main legitimate way is the one set apart by steady assurance.

Nonetheless, stopping is certainly not a one-size-fits-all idea. There are circumstances where stopping is an essential retreat, a fundamental stage towards a really encouraging future.

In the expert domain, the feeling of dread toward being named a slacker can keep people from chasing after their actual interests. The sunk expense paradox, where people keep putting resources into a choice or try due to the assets previously contributed, further convolutes matters. The thought of stopping as a disappointment is profoundly instilled, making it moving for people to break free from unfulfilling professions or adventures.

The apprehension about judgment likewise reaches out to connections. Whether a well established companionship or a marriage has lost its flash, the choice to stop is in many cases joined by cultural examination. The strain to adjust to cultural assumptions can eclipse the requirement for self-improvement and satisfaction. Breaking the chains of cultural assumptions is, in itself, a critical test that people should explore on their excursion to freedom.

In addition, the apprehension about the obscure can deaden. Stopping frequently implies venturing into a strange area, and the vulnerability that accompanies it very well may overpower. The security of the natural, regardless of whether it is smothering, can appear to be desirable over the likely difficulties of the unexplored world. This dread is a strong hindrance, keeping numerous from taking the jump towards a more true and satisfying life.

Stopping difficulties likewise include a renegotiation of personality. People frequently characterize themselves by their jobs in the public eye, be it as a devoted proficient, a caring accomplice, or a capable parent. Stopping can disturb these laid out characters, prompting a time of contemplation and redefinition. This cycle is fundamental for self-improvement however can be muddling and awkward.

The cultural accentuation on progress as a straight way further confuses the method involved with stopping. The possibility that achievement is a consequence of immovable responsibility and constant advancement can make a feeling of disgrace for the people who decide to stray from the recommended direction. Stopping difficulties this story, featuring that achievement is an emotional idea that must be characterized by the person.

On the other side, there are occasions where stopping is seen as a demonstration of strengthening. This is especially clear in developments upholding for taking care of oneself and emotional wellness. Perceiving when to move away from overpowering responsibilities or harmful conditions is viewed as a demonstration of solidarity. The story around stopping is developing, with a developing affirmation that it isn't inseparable from disappointment but instead a vital and fearless decision.

Stopping difficulties additionally reach out to the inward domain, where people wrestle with their own feelings of dread, frailties, and willful constraints. The brain, molded by cultural standards and individual encounters, can turn into an impressive impediment in the excursion to break free. Beating these psychological obstructions requires a profound comprehension of oneself and a guarantee to self-awareness.

Feeling of dread toward disappointment is a typical mental hindrance that people face while considering stopping. The apprehension that stopping is a confirmation of deficiency or a failure to succeed can incapacitate. Nonetheless, reevaluating disappointment as a learning a valuable open door and a venturing stone towards development can mitigate this trepidation. Stopping, in this specific circumstance, turns into a cognizant decision to divert one's endeavors towards a more significant and satisfying way.

Self-question is another interior test that people should stand up to. The inward pundit, filled by cultural assumptions and previous encounters, can stir up misgivings about one's capacities and value. Defeating self-question requires developing self-empathy and a faith in one's innate worth. Stopping turns into a demonstration of self-confirmation, a statement that one merits a daily existence lined up with their true self.

Notwithstanding mental obstructions, the profound cost of stopping difficulties is huge. Pain, responsibility, and a feeling of misfortune frequently go with the choice to stop. Whether it's the passing of a task, a relationship, or a recognizable lifestyle, the personal disturbance can be significant. People might wrestle with sensations of disappointment and frustration, further exacerbated by cultural assumptions.

Exploring the close to home scene of stopping requires flexibility and a readiness to defy awkward feelings. Lamenting the deficiency of the recognizable is a characteristic piece of the interaction, yet it shouldn't eclipse the potential for fresh starts. Embracing the full range of feelings, from pity to trust, is fundamental for mending and pushing ahead.

Stopping difficulties additionally feature the significance of emotionally supportive networks. Whether it's companions, family, or expert instructors, having an organization of people who comprehend and approve the choice to stop can have a massive effect. The excursion to break liberated from binds isn't intended to be attempted alone. The aggregate insight and consolation of a strong local area can give the strength expected to deal with difficulties directly.

The most common way of stopping difficulties frequently includes a time of reflection and self-disclosure. People might scrutinize their qualities, needs, and long-held convictions. This excursion of self-investigation is a fundamental piece of self-improvement and can prompt a more legitimate and deliberate life. Stopping turns into an impetus for positive change, an entryway to a future lined up with one's actual self.

Besides, stopping difficulties the cultural story of progress as an objective. Achievement, in the conventional sense, is in many cases depicted as a decent point that one should endeavor to reach. Stopping disturbs this direct story, underlining that achievement is a dynamic and developing idea. It's anything but an objective yet a ceaseless excursion of self-revelation, development, and transformation.

The idea of stopping difficulties additionally reaches out to cultural designs and standards that sustain disparity and unfairness. Developments for social change frequently include people and networks stopping complicity with severe frameworks. This type of stopping is an aggregate demonstration of obstruction, a refusal to be limited by chains of fundamental separation. It requires boldness, fortitude, and a promise to destroying unreasonable designs.

In the domain of self-improvement, stopping difficulties can be seen as a type of self-reevaluation. The choice to stop means a cognizant decision to shed old personalities and embrace the potential for change. This interaction isn't direct or unsurprising; it includes a ceaseless pattern of reflection, activity, and transformation. Stopping turns into a device for chiseling a daily existence that lines up with one's developing qualities and yearnings.

The excursion of stopping difficulties isn't without its mishaps and snapshots of uncertainty. The outer and interior opposition looked during this interaction can be imposing. Notwithstanding, unequivocally these difficulties add to the profundity and extravagance of the excursion. Every snag turns into a chance for learning, flexibility, and self-revelation.

At last, breaking the chains through stopping difficulties is a profoundly private and extraordinary excursion. It is an affirmation that life is excessively valuable to be lived in congruity with outside assumptions or in the grip of purposeful constraints.

Stopping, when drawn nearer with aim and mindfulness, turns into a useful asset for shaping a day to day existence that is significant, legitimate, and lined up with one's actual self.

As people explore the intricacies of stopping difficulties, developing an outlook of self-compassion is fundamental. The excursion isn't about flawlessness however about the ability to embrace weakness and blemish. Stopping turns into a gutsy demonstration of self esteem, a promise to respecting one's true necessities and yearnings.

All in all, breaking the chains through stopping difficulties is a complex and gutsy undertaking. It includes perceiving when the ongoing way no longer serves one's prosperity and daring to produce another direction. The cultural discernments encompassing stopping as a disappointment or shortcoming should be reconsidered, and the story reevaluated to recognize the strength and flexibility intrinsic in pursuing striking decisions.

The excursion of stopping difficulties incorporates proficient pursuits, connections, addictions, and cultural designs. It expects people to go up against outer assumptions, interior hindrances, and the profound cost of giving up. Through this interaction, people have the chance to reclassify achievement, embrace self-improvement, and add to more extensive developments for social change.

Stopping difficulties are not a one-time occasion but rather a ceaseless and dynamic interaction. It includes a continuous obligation to self-disclosure, variation, and the quest for a day to day existence that is true and satisfying. The chains that tight spot might be imposing, however the excursion of stopping moves is a demonstration of the unstoppable human soul and its ability for change.

### 6.1 Analysis of various cessation methods

The quest for stopping, whether it be stopping smoking, conquering dependence, or bringing an end to liberated from disastrous propensities, is a complex and profoundly private excursion. Various suspension strategies exist, each intended to address explicit difficulties and conditions. In this complete examination, we will investigate a scope of suspension strategies, looking at their viability, fundamental standards, and likely advantages and downsides.

One of the most well-known end strategies is pure and simple, a term that suggests stopping unexpectedly without steady decrease or outside helps. Pure and simple is in many cases seen as a trial of self discipline, requesting an unequivocal end from the propensity. While certain people effectively quit out of the blue, the methodology isn't without challenges. The unexpected discontinuance can prompt serious withdrawal side effects, making it a troublesome technique for those with solid conditions.

Nicotine substitution treatment (NRT) is another generally utilized discontinuance technique, especially for people endeavoring to stop smoking. NRT includes the utilization of nicotine-containing items, like patches, gum, capsules, or nasal splashes, to diminish nicotine reliance step by step. By giving controlled portions of nicotine, NRT means to ease withdrawal side effects while permitting people to acclimate to diminished nicotine levels. While NRT has demonstrated viable for the overwhelming majority, achievement rates shift, and a few people might battle with the lengthy utilization of nicotine items.

Pharmacological intercessions, for example, physician recommended meds, offer one more road for stopping. Bupropion and varenicline are instances of drugs intended to help smoking discontinuance. Bupropion, a stimulant, decreases withdrawal side effects and desires, while varenicline targets nicotine receptors in the cerebrum, lessening the pleasurable impacts of smoking. These prescriptions can be viable, however they accompany expected secondary effects, and their appropriateness shifts in view of individual wellbeing profiles.

Conduct treatment assumes a critical part in numerous suspension programs. This approach centers around recognizing and adjusting the ways of behaving related with the propensity being referred to. Mental social treatment (CBT), for example, helps people perceive and change thought examples and ways of behaving that add to the propensity. Social treatment can be utilized related to other end techniques, tending to the mental parts of compulsion and advancing long haul conduct change.

Persuasive improvement treatment (MET) is one more conduct approach that expects to expand a person's inherent inspiration to stop. MET commonly includes customized criticism, objective setting, and investigation of the singular's uncertainty toward stopping. By improving inspiration and responsibility, MET tries to engage people to move toward end.

Care based approaches have acquired prominence lately as compelling apparatuses for stopping. Care includes developing attention to considerations, feelings, and sensations right now without judgment. Care based backslide counteraction (MBRP) consolidates customary backslide anticipation procedures with care strategies. By expanding mindfulness and acknowledgment, MBRP outfits people with abilities to adapt to desires and stressors, decreasing the gamble of backslide.

Hypnotherapy is another elective discontinuance strategy that spotlights on adjusting the singular's condition of cognizance to advance conduct change. During hypnotherapy meetings, people enter a casual state, making them more responsive to ideas pointed toward getting out from under the propensity. While some make progress with hypnotherapy, its viability changes, and logical proof supporting its adequacy is restricted.

Needle therapy, established in conventional Chinese medication, includes the addition of flimsy needles into explicit focuses on the body. Defenders of needle therapy for smoking suspension contend that it can decrease withdrawal side effects and desires. Be that as it may, research on the viability of needle therapy for stopping smoking is uncertain, for certain investigations recommending unobtrusive advantages while others find no huge contrast contrasted with farce needle therapy.

Versatile applications and advanced stages have arisen as present day devices for end support. These applications frequently give a blend of educational assets, following highlights, and intuitive components to help people in their stopping process. While the openness and comfort of computerized intercessions are engaging, their adequacy might differ, and not all people make supported progress utilizing these instruments.

Social help and gathering treatment assume fundamental parts in numerous discontinuance programs. The force of local area and shared encounters couldn't possibly be more significant. Bunch treatment meetings give a steady climate where people can transparently examine their battles, share survival methods, and celebrate triumphs.

Peer support, whether face to face or through web-based gatherings, cultivates a feeling of association and diminishes sensations of disconnection.

Fitting end techniques to individual inclinations and requirements is pivotal for progress. Customized or accuracy medication approaches consider factors like hereditary inclinations, psychological well-being status, and way of life contemplations to configuration designated mediations. By perceiving the remarkable difficulties every individual appearances, customized suspension systems plan to upgrade adequacy and work on long haul results.

The coordination of innovation and creative methodologies keeps on growing the scene of end techniques. Computer generated reality (VR) treatment, for instance, submerges people in reasonable situations where they work on survival methods and refusal abilities. VR can be especially compelling in tending to desires and triggers by giving a controlled and vivid climate for openness treatment.

Craftsmanship and innovative treatments offer an elective way to deal with conventional end techniques. Expressive expressions, like music, dance, and visual expressions, furnish people with source for self-articulation and close to home handling. Taking part in imaginative exercises can be an incredible asset for overseeing pressure, nervousness, and desires, adding to an all encompassing way to deal with stopping.

Ecological alterations address a frequently neglected part of discontinuance. Establishing a steady climate includes recognizing and addressing triggers that add to the propensity. This might incorporate rebuilding everyday schedules, keeping away from places related with the propensity, and enrolling the help of loved ones in keeping a sans smoke or compulsion free space.

Mix treatments, which include the concurrent utilization of different suspension strategies, are building up some forward movement as far reaching ways to deal with stopping. Consolidating pharmacotherapy with social intercessions, for example, addresses both the physiological and mental parts of fixation. The collaboration of various methodologies can upgrade viability and backing people in their journey to break liberated from the chains of compulsion.

Backslide anticipation procedures are vital to supporting long haul end. Understanding that difficulties might happen and creating survival techniques to explore these difficulties is vital. Backslide counteraction programs frequently incorporate continuous help, expertise building activities, and procedures for overseeing high-risk circumstances. By enabling people to expect and address possible traps, backslide avoidance improves the probability of supported achievement.

The adequacy of end techniques is innately connected to individual changeability.

Factors, for example, the degree of reliance, coinciding psychological well-being conditions, and by and large status to stop assume crucial parts in deciding the outcome of a specific methodology. Perceiving the assorted requirements of people is fundamental for fitting suspension intercessions and improving results.

The continuous advancement of end examination and intercessions highlights the powerful idea of dependence and stopping. Progresses in neuroscience, pharmacology, and social science add to the improvement of more designated and powerful suspension strategies. The combination of arising advancements and a more profound comprehension of the natural and mental underpinnings of dependence offer promising roads for future developments in discontinuance methodologies.

All in all, the examination of different discontinuance techniques uncovers an assorted scene of approaches pointed toward helping people in their excursion to stop smoking, conquer compulsion, or bring an end to liberated from disastrous propensities. From customary strategies like pure and simple and nicotine substitution treatment to imaginative methodologies, for example, computer generated reality treatment and inventive expressions mediations, people have a huge number of choices to browse in light of their extraordinary necessities and inclinations.

The adequacy of every end strategy is nuanced and affected by individual elements, featuring the significance of customized and comprehensive methodologies. Joining pharmacological intercessions with conduct treatment, consolidating care practices, and utilizing social help all add to a thorough methodology for breaking the chains of enslavement. As the field of suspension research keeps on propelling, the expectation is to refine and tailor mediations to boost achievement rates and backing people in accomplishing and keeping a daily existence liberated from the limitations of enslavement.

### 6.2 The psychological and physical hurdles of quitting

Stopping, whether it be breaking liberated from drugs, conquering disastrous propensities, or withdrawing from unsafe connections, is a complex excursion that includes defeating both mental and actual obstacles. The choice to stop frequently emerges from an acknowledgment that the present status is unreasonable, yet the way to freedom is laden with difficulties. This exposition digs into the many-sided exchange of mental and actual snags looked by people in their mission to break liberated from the chains that tight spot them.

Mentally, the choice to stop is much of the time joined by a blast of clashing feelings. The feeling of dread toward the obscure, the uneasiness of progress, and the nervousness about potential mishaps can make a psychological scene loaded up with vulnerability. The mental obstacles of stopping are well established in the anxiety toward misfortune — loss of the recognizable, loss of character, and the apparent loss of survival techniques.

One of the essential mental obstacles is the feeling of dread toward disappointment. Society, with its accentuation on progress and accomplishment, frequently depicts stopping as inseparable from surrendering or conceding rout. This discernment can weigh vigorously on people examining a critical life altering event, supporting the shame related with stopping. Conquering the anxiety toward disappointment requires a change in mentality — an acknowledgment that stopping can be a demonstration of boldness and self-protection as opposed to an admission to shortcoming.

Also, the mental difficulties of stopping are unpredictably attached to self-insight. People frequently characterize themselves by their propensities, connections, or jobs in the public eye. Stopping upsets these laid out characters, prompting a time of reflection and reconsideration. The subject of "Who am I without this propensity or relationship?" turns into a focal concern, and exploring this character shift can sincerely burden.

The anxiety toward judgment from others additionally poses a potential threat on the mental scene of stopping. Whether it's the judgment of companions, family, or society at large, the apparent examination can make a strong impediment. The longing for social acknowledgment and the anxiety toward being marked a loser can obstruct the choice to break liberated from destructive examples. Conquering this mental obstacle includes developing a healthy identity worth that isn't dependent upon outer approval.

Additionally, the mental obstacles stretch out to the domain of desires and triggers. The psyche, molded by tedious ways of behaving and affiliations, can make strong desires to participate in the natural propensity. Defeating these desires includes a cognizant work to oppose as well as a comprehension of the mental triggers that initiate the craving to enjoy. This mindfulness is pivotal for creating successful survival methods.

Hidden mental variables, like pressure, tension, and gloom, can likewise present huge difficulties to stopping. People frequently go to propensities or substances as survival strategies for profound trouble. Stopping requires resolving these fundamental issues, which might require remedial mediations or the improvement of option, better ways of dealing with stress. The interconnectedness of emotional well-being and habit-forming ways of behaving highlights the significance of a comprehensive way to deal with stopping.

As opposed to the mind boggling scene of mental obstacles, the actual difficulties of stopping are many times more substantial yet no less considerable. Reliance on substances like nicotine, liquor, or medications can prompt withdrawal side effects that reach from somewhat awkward to strongly troubling. Actual withdrawal side effects can incorporate cerebral pains, sickness, peevishness, sleep deprivation, and desires, making the most common way of stopping truly requesting.

Nicotine withdrawal, specifically, is known for its difficult side effects. The sudden end of nicotine admission can prompt a scope of physical and mental side effects ordinarily known as nicotine withdrawal condition. These side effects incorporate crabbiness, uneasiness, discouraged state of mind, expanded hunger, and trouble concentrating. The seriousness and length of withdrawal side effects change from one individual to another, further convoluting the stopping system.

Liquor withdrawal represents its own arrangement of actual difficulties. Side effects like quakes, perspiring, sickness, and even seizures can happen in people with liquor reliance who endeavor to suddenly stop. The gamble of extreme withdrawal side effects highlights the significance of looking for proficient clinical direction while stopping specific substances.

Past withdrawal side effects, the actual obstacles of stopping additionally remember the acclimation to changes for routine and way of life. Propensities, whether they include substance use or different ways of behaving, frequently become imbued in day to day existence. Stopping requires a rebuilding of these schedules, making a void that people should explore. This change period can be truly and intellectually debilitating, as people wrestle with the newness of an existence without the natural propensity.

Rest unsettling influences are a typical actual test during the stopping system. Whether it's nicotine, caffeine, or different substances influencing rest designs, people frequently experience disturbances in their rest quality and term while endeavoring to stop. The significance of supportive rest in general prosperity makes tending to these rest unsettling influences a pivotal part of the stopping venture.

The effect of stopping on actual wellbeing is nuanced. While the demonstration of stopping is for the most part connected with long haul medical advantages, the quick consequence can be set apart by transitory uneasiness. This uneasiness might appear as weight gain, changes in hunger, or variances in energy levels. Understanding and tolerating these momentary changes are fundamental for people exploring the actual obstacles of stopping.

At times, people might confront existing together medical issue that entangle the stopping system. Constant torment, for instance, can be both a physical and mental boundary to stopping, as people might depend on substances for torment the board. The joining of medical care experts and custom-made end plans becomes vital in tending to the crossing point of actual wellbeing and habit-forming ways of behaving.

The polarity among mental and actual obstacles isn't outright; rather, it mirrors the multifaceted transaction among brain and body in the stopping venture. The brain body association is apparent in peculiarities, for example, stress-prompted desires, where mental stressors trigger actual reactions that drive people toward their natural propensities. Perceiving and tending to this brain body interchange is fundamental for creating extensive end systems.

Defeating the mental and actual obstacles of stopping requires an all encompassing and individualized approach. Social treatments, like mental conduct treatment (CBT) and inspirational improvement treatment (MET), address the mental parts of dependence by assisting people with changing idea designs, upgrade inspiration, and foster adapting abilities. These restorative methodologies are in many cases necessary parts of thorough suspension programs.

The utilization of pharmacotherapy, including nicotine substitution treatment (NRT) and doctor prescribed drugs, addresses the actual parts of withdrawal. NRT gives controlled dosages of nicotine to mitigate desires, while drugs like bupropion and varenicline focus on the mind's receptors to lessen withdrawal side effects and the pleasurable impacts of substances. The mix of social and pharmacological mediations improves the probability of effective stopping.

Care based approaches, for example, care based backslide counteraction (MBRP), offer a scaffold between the mental and actual domains of stopping. By developing consciousness of contemplations, feelings, and actual sensations, people foster a more prominent comprehension of the psyche body association. Care methods give devices to overseeing desires, stress, and the general inconvenience related with stopping.

Actual work and exercise assume a significant part in tending to both the mental and actual obstacles of stopping. Practice has been displayed to lessen pressure, further develop state of mind, and alleviate withdrawal side effects. Moreover, captivating in normal actual work can assist people with overseeing weight changes related with stopping and add to a general feeling of prosperity.

Dietary mediations likewise structure a part of tending to actual difficulties during the stopping system. People might encounter changes in hunger and dietary examples, and keeping a reasonable and nutritious eating regimen can uphold generally well-being. Legitimate hydration is similarly significant, as it adds to actual prosperity and helps flush substances from the body.

Social help arises as a strong partner in defeating the mental and actual obstacles of stopping. The feeling of local area, understanding, and shared encounters presented by help gatherings and advising can altogether influence a singular's capacity to explore the difficulties of stopping. Peer support cultivates a feeling of association, diminishing sensations of detachment and giving commonsense experiences into the stopping venture.

Tending to the mental and actual obstacles of stopping requires a supported and cooperative exertion. Medical services experts, including doctors, clinicians, and habit trained professionals, assume essential parts in directing people through the stopping system. Fitting intercessions to individual necessities, offering continuous help, and addressing coinciding medical issue add to a more far reaching and successful way to deal with stopping.

### 6.3 Success stories of individuals who successfully quit smoking

The excursion of stopping smoking is an imposing test, however various people all over the planet have shown striking flexibility and assurance in effectively breaking liberated from the chains of tobacco dependence. These examples of overcoming adversity rouse others on their stopping process as well as feature the different ways people take to accomplish sans smoke lives. In looking at these examples of overcoming adversity, normal subjects of inspiration, emotionally supportive networks, survival methods, and self-awareness arise as key variables in the excursion to stop smoking.

One repeating subject in examples of overcoming adversity is the strong inspiration that drives people to stop smoking. Inspiration frequently comes from a longing to work on one's wellbeing, shield friends and family from handed-down cigarette smoke, or recapture command over one's life. Wellbeing related inspirations, like lessening the gamble of cardiovascular sickness, respiratory issues, and malignant growth, act as convincing motivations to set out on the difficult way of stopping. The acknowledgment that smoking unmistakably affects individual prosperity turns into a main impetus for change.

Family and relational connections assume a critical part in the examples of overcoming adversity of numerous people who quit smoking. The longing to be available for family achievements, for example, seeing youngsters grow up or becoming grandparents, fills in as a strong inspiration. The effect of smoking on relational peculiarities, combined with the wish to be a positive good example, frequently catalyzes the choice to stop. The help and consolation of relatives make a powerful starting point for the stopping venture.

Besides, examples of overcoming adversity much of the time highlight the significance of a solid emotionally supportive network. Whether it be family, companions, or care groups, having an organization of people who comprehend the difficulties of stopping is instrumental. The common encounters, consolation, and responsibility offered by a help framework contribute essentially to keeping up with inspiration during the high points and low points of the stopping system. Peer support frequently turns into a significant point of support in the excursion toward a sans smoke life.

People who effectively quit smoking much of the time utilize various survival techniques to explore desires and withdrawal side effects. Conduct procedures, for example, care and profound breathing activities, assist with overseeing pressure and divert contemplations from the inclination to smoke. Participating in proactive tasks, whether it be standard activity or leisure activities, gives a solid outlet to push and an interruption from desires. Creating elective survival techniques turns into a focal part of the stopping venture.

Numerous examples of overcoming adversity feature the utilization of nicotine substitution treatment (NRT) as an instrument to oversee withdrawal side effects. NRT, as patches, gum, tablets, or nasal showers, assists individuals with steadily decreasing their nicotine reliance. The controlled dosages of nicotine given by NRT reduce desires and add to the general outcome of the stopping system. Examples of overcoming adversity frequently stress the job of NRT as a feature of a thorough methodology that incorporates social and everyday reassurance.

The consolidation of innovation into the stopping venture is a striking element in present day examples of overcoming adversity. Portable applications, quitline administrations, and online networks offer people advantageous and available assets for help and direction. The intuitive elements of these advanced apparatuses, like following advancement, defining objectives, and getting persuasive messages, add to the feeling of strengthening and responsibility in the stopping system. Examples of overcoming adversity much of the time feature the positive effect of innovation in giving extra layers of help.

Self-improvement and the improvement of a positive mentality arise as extraordinary components in the examples of overcoming adversity of the people who quit smoking. The stopping venture frequently includes a significant change in self-discernment — from a smoker to a non-smoker. People portray a freshly discovered feeling of strengthening, expanded confidence, and an increased familiarity with their own flexibility. The capacity to beat difficulties turns into a wellspring of pride and further persuades people to keep up with their sans smoke status.

A consistent idea in examples of overcoming adversity is the acknowledgment of difficulties as learning potential open doors as opposed to disappointments. Backslides are recognized as a component of the stopping system, and people who effectively quit smoking frequently share bits of knowledge acquired from their own encounters with impermanent mishaps. The capacity to gain from backslides, recognize sets off, and change procedures adds to long haul achievement. Examples of overcoming adversity feature the significance of flexibility and versatility in beating the difficulties of stopping.

The effect of monetary contemplations is one more feature every now and again referenced in examples of overcoming adversity. The acknowledgment of the significant expense of smoking — both as far as the immediate cost of cigarettes and potential medical services costs — turns into a rousing variable for some people to stop. The possibility of setting aside cash and diverting it toward additional satisfying pursuits fills in as an unmistakable and compensating part of the stopping venture.

Ecological and way of life changes are in many cases necessary parts of examples of overcoming adversity. Making a sans smoke living space, keeping away from triggers, and embracing better propensities add to the general outcome of stopping smoking. Examples of overcoming adversity every now and again accentuate the significance of effectively molding one's current circumstance to help the objective of outstanding sans smoke. Way of life changes, remembering upgrades for diet and expanded actual work, become positive anchors in the excursion to better wellbeing.

The festival of achievements and accomplishments, both little and huge, is a repetitive subject in examples of overcoming adversity. Recognizing the headway made, whether it be seven days, a month, or a year without smoking, builds up the feeling of achievement and fills in as encouraging feedback. Examples of overcoming adversity frequently underscore the significance of perceiving and commending these achievements to support inspiration and responsibility.

The assorted pathways to outcome in stopping smoking highlight the individualized idea of the stopping venture. While specific subjects, like inspiration, support, survival techniques, and self-awareness, wind through these accounts, the exceptional conditions and points of view of every individual add to a rich embroidery of stories. Examples of overcoming adversity stress that there is nobody size-fits-all way to deal with stopping; rather, the excursion is a dynamic and individual interaction.

All in all, the examples of overcoming adversity of people who have stopped smoking act as strong tributes to the strength of the human soul. Spurred by wellbeing concerns, relational connections, and a longing for self-improvement, these people explore the mental and actual obstacles of stopping sincerely and diligence. Emotionally supportive networks, survival methods, and a positive outlook assume pivotal parts in the examples of overcoming adversity, showing that the stopping venture isn't just about defeating compulsion yet additionally about embracing a new and satisfying lifestyle. These accounts rouse and enlighten the bunch opportunities for the people who leave on their own excursion to break liberated from the chains of smoking.

The tales of people who have effectively stopped smoking are strong stories that enlighten the difficulties, wins, and individual changes that go with the excursion to a without smoke life. These accounts act as encouraging signs for those right now battling with tobacco fixation, showing that stopping isn't just imaginable however can likewise prompt significant positive changes in one's wellbeing, connections, and generally prosperity.

Inspiration arises as a focal subject in the examples of overcoming adversity of people who have stopped smoking. The impetuses for this inspiration differ generally, frequently established in a well established craving for better wellbeing. Numerous people share a typical acknowledgment that smoking is hindering to their actual prosperity, filling in as an essential inspiration to start the stopping system. Worries about lung wellbeing, cardiovascular dangers, and the general effect of smoking on future become strong main thrusts.

As far as some might be concerned, the inspiration to stop smoking is interwoven with a promise to shielding friends and family from the hurtful impacts of handed-down cigarette smoke. Guardians express a craving to be available for their kids' achievements and to set a positive model for the future. The effect of smoking on relational peculiarities turns into a strong inspiration, supporting the purpose to break liberated from the chains of enslavement.

Wellbeing related inspirations reach out past the actual domain to envelop mental and close to home prosperity. People who effectively quit smoking frequently depict enhancements in their psychological lucidity, profound flexibility, and generally speaking state of mind. The lightening of tension and stress, when veiled by the impermanent help given by cigarettes, turns into a critical positive result of the stopping venture. Examples of overcoming adversity regularly feature the interconnectedness of physical and emotional well-being in the journey for a sans smoke life.

The job of emotionally supportive networks arises as an ongoing idea in examples of overcoming adversity. Whether it be the consolation of relatives, the fellowship of companions who have likewise stopped, or the direction of care groups and guides, the presence of a vigorous encouraging group of people is a characterizing factor in the stopping venture. The common encounters, compassion, and responsibility offered by these help frameworks contribute fundamentally to a singular's capacity to explore the difficulties of stopping.

Support from medical services experts is many times instrumental in the examples of overcoming adversity of the people who quit smoking. Doctors, attendants, and habit experts assume critical parts in giving direction, endorsing prescriptions when fitting, and observing advancement. The coordination of clinical skill into the stopping system upgrades the probability of accomplishment, particularly when joined with social intercessions and customized end plans.

Survival techniques structure a basic part of examples of overcoming adversity, as people foster imaginative and powerful methods for overseeing desires and explore the close to home highs and lows of stopping. Conduct methods, like care and profound breathing activities, arise as significant apparatuses to divert considerations from the desire to smoke. Taking part in proactive tasks, whether it be standard activity or leisure activities, gives a solid outlet to stretch and an interruption from desires. Examples of overcoming adversity habitually highlight the significance of developing a different tool stash of methods for dealing with stress customized to individual necessities.

Nicotine substitution treatment (NRT) is in many cases refered to in examples of overcoming adversity as a supportive guide in overseeing withdrawal side effects. The controlled portions of nicotine given by NRT, as patches, gum, capsules, or nasal showers, ease desires and add to the general progress of the stopping system. Examples of overcoming adversity feature the essential utilization of NRT as a component of a thorough methodology that incorporates social help and way of life changes.

The joining of innovation into the stopping venture is a remarkable component in present day examples of overcoming adversity. Portable applications, quitline administrations, and online networks offer people helpful and available assets for help and direction. The intuitive highlights of these computerized apparatuses, for example, progress following, objective setting, and persuasive messages, add to the feeling of strengthening and responsibility in the stopping system. Examples of overcoming adversity every now and again feature the positive effect of innovation in giving extra layers of help.

Self-improvement and the advancement of a positive mentality arise as extraordinary components in the examples of overcoming adversity of the people who quit smoking. The stopping venture frequently includes a significant change in self-discernment — from a smoker to a non-smoker. People portray a newly discovered feeling of strengthening, expanded confidence, and an increased familiarity with their own versatility. The capacity to beat difficulties turns into a wellspring of pride and further propels people to keep up with their sans smoke status.

Mishaps and backslides are recognized as a component of the stopping system in examples of overcoming adversity, exhibiting the significance of flexibility and versatility. As opposed to survey backslides as disappointments, people who effectively quit smoking offer experiences acquired from transitory mishaps. Gaining from backslides, recognizing triggers, and changing techniques in light of individual encounters add to long haul achievement. Examples of overcoming adversity feature the iterative idea of the stopping venture and the capacity to persist notwithstanding difficulties.

Monetary contemplations frequently act as extra inspiration in examples of overcoming adversity. The combined expense of smoking — both as far as the immediate cost of cigarettes and potential medical services costs — turns into a convincing motivation to stop. The possibility of setting aside cash and diverting it toward additional satisfying pursuits fills in as an unmistakable and compensating part of the stopping venture. Examples of overcoming adversity habitually underline the positive effect of stopping on monetary prosperity.

Ecological and way of life changes are vital parts of examples of overcoming adversity. Making a sans smoke living space, keeping away from triggers, and embracing better propensities add to the general outcome of stopping smoking. Examples of overcoming adversity every now and again stress the significance of effectively forming one's current circumstance to help the objective of residual without smoke. Way of life changes, remembering enhancements for diet and expanded active work, become positive anchors in the excursion to better wellbeing.

Commending achievements and accomplishments, both little and huge, is a repetitive subject in examples of overcoming adversity. Recognizing progress, whether it be seven days, a month, or a year without smoking, builds up the feeling of achievement and fills in as encouraging feedback.

Examples of overcoming adversity frequently underline the significance of perceiving and praising these achievements to support inspiration and responsibility all through the stopping venture.

The assorted pathways to progress in stopping smoking highlight the individualized idea of the excursion. While specific subjects, like inspiration, support, survival methods, and self-awareness, wind through these accounts, the novel conditions and viewpoints of every individual add to a rich embroidery of stories. Examples of overcoming adversity underscore that there is nobody size-fits-all way to deal with stopping; rather, the excursion is a dynamic and individual interaction.

Taking everything into account, the examples of overcoming adversity of people who have stopped smoking act as strong tributes to the versatility of the human soul. Persuaded by wellbeing concerns, relational connections, and a craving for self-improvement, these people explore the mental and actual obstacles of stopping sincerely and steadiness. Emotionally supportive networks, survival methods, and a positive outlook assume pivotal parts in the examples of overcoming adversity, showing that the stopping venture isn't just about conquering compulsion yet in addition about embracing a new and satisfying lifestyle. These accounts rouse and enlighten the bunch opportunities for the individuals who leave on their own excursion to break liberated from the chains of smoking.

# Chapter 7

### The Paradoxical Pleasure

In the maze of human experience, the perplexing idea of delight winds around an embroidery that rises above ordinary comprehension. The human mind is a complicated scene, where delight frequently arises as a conundrum, resisting oversimplified order. A complex jewel refracts horde tints, every feature mirroring the exchange of science, brain research, and culture. The dumbfounding joy that traps the human spirit is a bewildering dance among joy and misery, want and limitation, freedom and imprisonment.

Joy, in its substance, is a base power that courses through the veins of presence. From the delicate bit of a friend or family member to the epicurean enjoyments of extravagance, joy shapes our insights and varieties the material of our lives. However, this apparently direct idea is loaded with logical inconsistencies that puzzle our comprehension. The oddity lies in the many-sided joining of delight with its shadowy partner, torment. It is in the acknowledgment that joy and torment are not fundamentally unrelated yet rather two of a kind, each upgrading the power of the other.

One can't completely see the value in the delight of joy without the differentiating setting of torment. The sharp edges of distress emphasize the sweet tune of bliss. This perplexing dance of joy and torment is profoundly implanted in the human experience, a piercing sign of the fragile equilibrium that characterizes our close to home scene. It is through the pot of misfortune that the real essence of joy is uncovered, arising like a phoenix from the remains of depression.

The Catch 22 reaches out past the domain of feelings to the actual center of human science. The libertine quest for joy is unpredictably connected with the multifaceted hardware of the cerebrum, where synapses and chemicals organize the ensemble of sensation. Dopamine, the synapse ordinarily connected with delight, turns into a blade that cuts both ways, driving us to look for satisfaction while likewise delivering us defenseless against the impulses of fixation. The delight looking for pathways in the mind are a demonstration of the transformative foundations of this oddity, where the quest for joy was once an endurance system guaranteeing the proliferation of the species.

However, in the complicated embroidery of current presence, the conundrum of joy takes on new aspects. The quest for joy turns into a nuanced dance between moment satisfaction and long haul satisfaction. In a world immersed with improvements, the enticement of prompt joy frequently overshadows the subtler delights that require persistence and determination. The oddity lies in the strain between the vaporous bliss existing apart from everything else and the persevering through satisfaction that comes from developing significant associations and seeking after a reason driven life.

The perplexing idea of delight is likewise apparent in the domains of want and restriction. The indulgent motivations that drive us to look for delight conflict with the cultural standards and moral codes that endorse control and self-restraint. The quest for joy turns into a tightrope stroll between the freeing leave of want and the controlling power of cultural assumptions. This pressure among extravagance and restriction shapes the ethical texture of social orders and people, leading to an intricate interchange of values and indecencies.

At the core of the confusing joy is the duality of freedom and bondage. The quest for delight is much of the time seen as a mission for freedom from the requirements of the real world, a brief break into a domain of uplifted sensation and leave. However, oddly, this very pursuit can turn into a type of imprisonment, capturing people in the snare of enslavement and overabundance. The freeing power of joy changes into a limiting chain, and the quest for joy turns into a Sisyphean battle against the shackles of one's own cravings.

In the domain of style, the Catch 22 of delight is apparent in the juxtaposition of excellence and rot. The charm of tasteful delight lies in the wonderful concordance of structure and capability, a brief snapshot of flawlessness that rises above the desolates of time.

However, this very magnificence is vaporous, dependent upon the unyielding walk of rot. The mystery lies in the synchronous festival of the transient and the everlasting, the delight got from excellence touched with the consciousness of its unavoidable death.

The perplexing joy is a repetitive theme in the embroidery of human connections. The euphoria of adoration is indistinguishable from the weakness of disaster. The closeness that ties spirits together is a sensitive dance between the joy of association and the aggravation of partition. The conundrum is in the acknowledgment that adoration, with all its delights and distresses, is a fundamental piece of the human experience, a power that rises above the limits of existence.

In the domain of otherworldliness, the oddity of delight takes on a significant aspect. The quest for profound edification is much of the time outlined as an excursion towards greatness, a journey to transcend the vaporous joys of the material world. However, strangely, numerous otherworldly customs perceive the characteristic worth of the body and the tangible experience as vehicles for divine acknowledgment. The joy got from otherworldly practices turns into a method for accomplishing a higher condition of cognizance, a confusing association of the material and the extraordinary.

The dumbfounding delight is likewise laced with the idea of debauchery, the way of thinking that sets joy as the most noteworthy great. The epicurean quest for joy, frequently connected with overabundance and guilty pleasure, turns into a landmark of clashing qualities. The delight searcher is conflicted between the quest for sure fire satisfaction and the consciousness of the expected outcomes. The decadent mystery lies in the pressure between the quest for delight for the wellbeing of its own and the acknowledgment of the requirement for equilibrium and balance.

In the domain of imagination, the conundrum of joy appears in the strain among motivation and discipline. The innovative flow is a sensitive dance between the unconstrained joy of motivation and the trained work of carrying thoughts to completion. The joy of creation is indistinguishable from the aggravation of imaginative battle, and the Catch 22 lies in the capacity to explore the back and forth movement of the imaginative excursion.

The confusing joy stretches out to the space of scholarly pursuits, where the journey for information is both a wellspring of enjoyment and a weight. The joy of revelation is tempered by the familiarity with the tremendous region of the unexplored world. The quest for scholarly joy turns into a confusing dance between the elation of understanding and the modesty notwithstanding the boundless secrets that escape perception.

With regards to cultural designs, the mystery of joy is reflected in the strain between individual longings and aggregate prosperity. The quest for individual delight frequently comes to the detriment of social concordance and natural manageability.

The mystery lies in the acknowledgment that unrestrained debauchery can sabotage the actual underpinnings of cultural attachment, requiring a sensitive harmony between individual opportunities and aggregate liability.

The dumbfounding joy is a subject that resonates through the chronicles of writing and reasoning. It finds articulation in the appalling stories of characters whose quest for joy prompts their defeat, as well as in the philosophical thoughts on the idea of bliss and the human condition. The incredible works of writing and reasoning wrestle with the inborn inconsistencies of joy, offering bits of knowledge that reverberate across societies and ages.

As the woven artwork of the incomprehensible joy unfurls, it becomes clear that this perplexing power is an essential piece of the human experience. A power shapes our discernments, drives our activities, and tones the embroidery of our lives. The Catch 22 lies in the multifaceted transaction of delight and agony, want and restriction, freedom and imprisonment. A dance rises above the limits of individual experience, winding around an ongoing idea that ties mankind in its aggregate quest for importance and satisfaction.

In the perplexing delight, we find the substance of being human — a mind boggling embroidery of feelings, wants, and encounters that challenge simple order. An update life's process is definitely not a straight way however a complex labyrinth where joy and torment, satisfaction and distress, are inseparably interwoven. The oddity welcomes us to embrace the inconsistencies, to explore the intricacies with elegance and versatility, and to track down importance in the many-sided dance of joy that shapes the human spirit.

All in all, the confusing joy is a spellbinding peculiarity that rises above the limits of individual experience, winding around a consistent idea that ties humankind in its aggregate quest for significance and satisfaction. This diverse jewel, with its mind boggling interaction of delight and torment, want and restriction, freedom and imprisonment, is a demonstration of the intricacy of the human experience. From the domains of science and brain research to the areas of connections, feel, otherworldliness, and cultural designs, the conundrum of joy appears in horde structures, forming the embroidery of human life.

As we explore the maze of life, the dumbfounding delight welcomes us to embrace the inconsistencies, to perceive the fragile equilibrium that characterizes our profound scene. It moves us to rise above oversimplified thoughts of joy and agony, welcoming us to investigate the nuanced dance between prompt satisfaction and persevering through satisfaction. In this investigation, we might find a more profound comprehension of ourselves and the unpredictable embroidery of the human experience, finding significance in the confusing joy that characterizes our excursion through the perplexing labyrinth of existence.

### 7.1 Examining the perceived pleasures of smoking

The demonstration of smoking, with its surging crest of smoke and cadenced inward breaths, has for some time been interlaced with a complicated trap of insights, ceremonies, and perplexing delights. Inspecting the apparent delights of smoking requires a nuanced investigation that goes past the superficial comprehension of a simple propensity. It digs into the mental, social, and social aspects that shape the smoker's insight, disentangling an embroidery of joy that is both profoundly private and unpredictably associated with more extensive cultural builds.

At the core of the apparent delights of smoking is the psychoactive substance nicotine, a strong alkaloid tracked down in tobacco. Nicotine, with its capacity to invigorate the arrival of synapses, for example, dopamine, assumes a focal part in causing a pleasurable situation for the smoker. The prompt impacts of nicotine, including expanded readiness and a feeling of unwinding, add to the charm of smoking. This pharmacological angle shapes the underpinning of the delight got from the demonstration.

Notwithstanding, the apparent joys of smoking stretch out a long ways past the physiological impacts of nicotine. Smoking is much of the time implanted in ceremonies and schedules, turning into a representative demonstration that conveys individual and social importance. The demonstration of lighting a cigarette, attracting the principal inward breath, and breathing out a crest of smoke can be a ceremonial encounter that intersperses snapshots of examination, social connection, or stress help. These ceremonies give a feeling of construction and commonality, adding layers of importance to the demonstration of smoking past its compound impacts.

The social component of smoking further enhances its apparent joys. Smoking has generally been a collective movement, cultivating a feeling of fellowship among people who share the custom. From the smoke-occupied private cabins of social clubs to the relaxed trades during a smoke break, the demonstration of smoking frequently fills in as a social paste, working with associations and discussions. The common experience of smoking makes a feeling of having a place and local area, upgrading the delight got from the demonstration.

The formal and social parts of smoking are entwined with social portrayals that shape the view of smoking as an image of disobedience, refinement, or recreation. The symbolism of the solitary renegade with a cigarette hanging from their lips or the glitzy Hollywood diva carefully holding a cigarette holder has added to the romanticization of smoking. These social portrayals implant smoking with undertones of opportunity, charm, and a specific persona, upgrading the apparent joys related with the demonstration.

However, analyzing the apparent joys of smoking requires recognizing the oddities that underlie this intricate way of behaving. Smoking, regardless of its apparent delights, is inseparably connected to a bunch of wellbeing gambles. The demonstration of breathing in the harmful parts of tobacco smoke is a significant supporter of different illnesses, including cellular breakdown in the lungs, coronary illness, and respiratory problems. The joy got from smoking exists in strain with the information on these wellbeing dangers, making a conundrum that people wrestle with as they explore their smoking propensities.

The Catch 22 is additionally intensified by the habit-forming nature of nicotine. What might start as a pleasurable encounter can rapidly change into an impulsive propensity as the body fosters a reliance on nicotine. The underlying joys of smoking become snared with the battle to fulfill the desires, prompting a pattern of habit that is hard to break. The apparent joys of smoking, established in the transaction of custom, socialization, and social imagery, become enmeshed with the physiological reliance on nicotine, making a perplexing embroidery that is trying to unwind.

Looking at the apparent joys of smoking likewise requires a more critical glance at the job of pressure and survival strategies in the smoker's insight. For some people, smoking fills in as a type of self-medicine, offering a fleeting getaway from the tensions of day to day existence. The demonstration of smoking turns into a ritualized reaction to push, giving a short break from uneasiness and pressure. In this specific situation, the apparent joy of smoking is intently attached to its capability as a survival strategy, a device for dealing with the burdens and kinds of presence.

The mental part of smoking as a survival strategy is interlaced with the tangible delights related with the demonstration. The material impression of holding a cigarette, the musical inward breaths, and the tactile criticism of breathing out smoke make a multisensory experience that connects with the smoker on an instinctive level.

This tangible commitment adds to the apparent delight of smoking, offering a tactile break that supplements the mental advantages of pressure help.

The assessment of the apparent joys of smoking is deficient disregarding the job of showcasing and promoting in forming the smoker's insight. Tobacco organizations have long grasped the force of picture and marking in developing the appeal of smoking. From notable logos to painstakingly created promoting efforts, the tobacco business has attempted to connect smoking with subjects of resistance, refinement, and social association. The cautiously organized symbolism adds to the development of smoking as a direction for living, upgrading the apparent joys related with the demonstration.

The standardization of smoking through promoting reaches out to the depiction of smoking in mainstream society. Motion pictures, network shows, and different types of media frequently portray smoking as an everyday and socially OK way of behaving.

This standardization adds to the support of smoking as a pleasurable and ordinary movement, further inserting it into the texture of cultural standards. The apparent joys of smoking, as formed by advertising and media, become interwoven with more extensive social stories that impact individual insights and ways of behaving.

Looking at the apparent joys of smoking likewise requires a thought of the job of individual organization and independence. People take part in smoking for various reasons, and the apparent joys related with the demonstration are emotional and setting subordinate. While cultural and social variables assume a huge part, the independence of the person in deciding to smoke or stop can't be ignored. Understanding the apparent delights of smoking requires recognizing the organization of smokers and perceiving the variables that impact their choices.

With regards to smoking suspension endeavors, the assessment of seen joys turns into an essential part of planning compelling mediations. Essentially featuring the wellbeing dangers of smoking may not be adequate to address the mind boggling trap of delights, ceremonies, and social elements that underlie the way of behaving. Fruitful smoking discontinuance programs should consider the complex idea of the apparent delights related with smoking, offering elective survival techniques, support designs, and methodologies for breaking the pattern of dependence.

All in all, looking at the apparent joys of smoking divulges a rich embroidery of encounters that stretch out past the pharmacological impacts of nicotine. The demonstration of smoking is woven into the texture of customs, social collaborations, and social imagery, making a mind boggling exchange of joys that is both individual and cultural. The charm of smoking is well established in the tangible commitment, the mental advantages of pressure help, and the shared perspectives that add to a feeling of having a place.

However, this embroidery of delights isn't without its Catch 22s. The wellbeing gambles and habit-forming nature of smoking cast a shadow over the apparent delights, making a pressure that people should explore as they wrestle with their smoking propensities. The assessment of seen delights likewise exposes the job of showcasing and social stories in forming the smoker's insight, affecting discernments and ways of behaving on both individual and cultural levels.

Eventually, understanding the apparent joys of smoking is a multi-layered try that requires a comprehensive methodology. It requires an investigation of the mental, social, and social aspects that add to the complicated snare of delights related with smoking. In disentangling this embroidery, specialists, policymakers, and general wellbeing experts can foster more far reaching techniques for smoking end, recognizing the independence of people while tending to the diverse idea of the apparent joys that underlie this profoundly imbued conduct.

### 7.2 Cultural and social aspects of smoking as a social activity

Smoking, past its singular wellbeing suggestions, is profoundly interlaced with social and social elements, frequently working as an intricate social movement. Looking at the social and social parts of smoking reveals an embroidery woven with customs, images, and public encounters that rise above the actual demonstration. From old customs to current group environments, smoking plays played different parts in molding social cooperations, character, and cultural standards.

Social points of view on smoking change broadly across various social orders and verifiable periods. In certain societies, smoking has been ritualized as a sacrosanct or formal demonstration, representing profound association, soul changing experiences, or contributions to divinities. The utilization of tobacco in native societies, for example, is in many cases well established in stately practices that stretch out past individual delight to mutual and otherworldly aspects. Inspecting these social subtleties gives a more profound comprehension of how smoking has been incorporated into the texture of human social orders, reflecting convictions, values, and customs.

In additional contemporary settings, smoking has developed into a complex social movement, frequently filling in for the purpose of association, unwinding, and articulation. Social smoking, described by the demonstration of smoking in gatherings or group environments, is a sign of how the social and social parts of smoking add to its pervasiveness. The common idea of smoking cultivates a feeling of kinship and having a place, making shared encounters and ceremonies that tight spot people together.

The social meaning of smoking is likewise clear in the emblematic implications ascribed to cigarettes and other tobacco items. The demonstration of sharing a cigarette can be a token of kinship, trust, or closeness. Lighting a cigarette in a group environment can flag a change, whether it destroy a feast, the start of a discussion, or a snapshot of consideration. The emblematic force of smoking reaches out to the stuff related with it, from rich cigarette holders to luxurious lines, each conveying its own social undertones.

The social and social parts of smoking are complicatedly connected to ideas of character and self-articulation. Smoking can turn into a marker of character, a way for people to fall in line with specific subcultures, ways of life, or defiant philosophies. The reception of smoking as a social practice is frequently attached to thoughts of opportunity, refinement, or rebelliousness, sustained by social portrayals in media and mainstream society. The smoker, in this unique situation, may see themselves as a component of a bigger story, embracing the social and social aspects that smoking bears.

Group environments frequently assume a vital part in forming smoking ways of behaving. Whether in bistros, bars, or assigned smoking regions, the demonstration of smoking is frequently entwined with shared spaces where people meet up. These conditions give a background to social cooperations, building up the public idea of smoking. Smoking turns into a social ointment, working with discussions, facilitating strains, and encouraging associations among people who participate in this common movement.

The standardization of smoking inside groups of friends is a urgent part of its social and social aspects. As people notice their companions taking part in smoking, it turns into a standardized way of behaving, building up the social worthiness of the demonstration. This standardization is additionally propagated by the depiction of smoking in media, where characters frequently smoke in friendly circumstances, adding to the social content that partners smoking with brotherhood and amiability.

The social part of smoking isn't restricted to casual get-togethers however stretches out to additional formalized occasions and ceremonies. The smoking of stogies, for instance, is frequently connected with celebratory events like weddings, births, or business triumphs. The social and social imagery of stogie smoking in such settings goes past the actual demonstration, turning into a ritualized articulation of satisfaction, accomplishment, or holding. Stogies, in these occasions, act as social relics that mark critical minutes in the aggregate existence of a local area.

Inspecting the social and social parts of smoking likewise requires an investigation of gendered aspects. By and large, smoking has been gendered, with unmistakable social and social implications ascribed to male and female smokers. The relationship of smoking with ideas of manliness or womanliness has molded the manners by which people explore their characters inside friendly settings. The breaking of orientation standards, with ladies embracing smoking in additional critical numbers during the twentieth 100 years, addresses a change in social and social impression of smoking and orientation.

Smoking has been a subject of social study and activism, especially concerning its effect on minimized networks. The tobacco business has been censured for focusing on unambiguous socioeconomics, including racial and ethnic gatherings, adding to wellbeing incongruities. Inspecting the social and social parts of smoking includes recognizing the multifacetedness of these elements, perceiving how social, social, and financial variables converge to impact smoking ways of behaving and results.

The social and social parts of smoking reach out to the domain of writing and human expression. From notorious pictures of craftsmen with cigarettes close by to artistic stories that mesh smoking into the texture of characters' lives, the social portrayals of smoking in imaginative works add to its representative power.

The demonstration of smoking in writing, film, and craftsmanship frequently fills in as a similitude, representing defiance, existential tension, or a quest for significance.

These social portrayals shape and reflect cultural mentalities toward smoking, affecting the way things are seen and experienced.

The assessment of the social and social parts of smoking likewise requires an investigation of against smoking efforts and general wellbeing drives. Endeavors to denormalize smoking, especially openly spaces, have expected to move cultural perspectives and ways of behaving. The execution of sans smoke strategies in different settings mirrors a more extensive social shift away from normalizing smoking in broad daylight. Understanding the social and social components of smoking is vital for planning successful general wellbeing mediations that address the mind boggling interchange of social standards, social elements, and individual ways of behaving.

Social and social factors likewise assume a huge part in smoking commencement among youngsters. The impact of companions, family, and cultural standards shapes youths' view of smoking. Looking at the social and social parts of smoking with regards to youth commencement includes understanding the job of publicizing, peer strain, and social acknowledgment in forming youthful people's perspectives toward smoking. Successful anticipation systems should consider the social and social aspects that add to smoking inception among the adolescent.

All in all, the social and social parts of smoking are a rich and complex embroidery that winds through the texture of human social orders. From antiquated ceremonies to present day group environments, smoking plays played assorted parts in molding common encounters, character, and cultural standards. The social meaning of smoking is reflected in ceremonies, images, and shared spaces where people meet up. The social part of smoking reaches out to both casual get-togethers and formalized occasions, filling in as a social oil that works with associations among people.

Social portrayals of smoking in media and mainstream society add to the standardization of smoking, sustaining social scripts that partner smoking with fellowship and friendliness. Gendered aspects of smoking uncover how social and social implications have been generally credited to male and female smokers. Scrutinizes of the tobacco business feature the multifacetedness of social, social, and monetary variables that impact smoking ways of behaving and wellbeing results.

Understanding the social and social parts of smoking is urgent for creating extensive general wellbeing intercessions and hostile to smoking efforts. Endeavors to denormalize smoking in broad daylight spaces and forestall youth commencement should think about the mind boggling transaction of social standards, social elements, and individual ways of behaving.

As social orders keep on advancing, so too will the social and social elements of smoking, molding and reflecting more extensive perspectives toward this mind boggling and diverse social movement.

### 7.3 The role of stress relief and relaxation in smoking behavior

The perplexing connection between stress help, unwinding, and smoking conduct shapes an intricate nexus that has enthralled specialists, wellbeing experts, and people the same. Analyzing the job of pressure help and unwinding in smoking way of behaving requires digging into the mental, physiological, and sociocultural aspects that add to the entwined idea of these components. While smoking is in many cases seen as a survival technique for stress, the elements are multi-layered, and a nuanced investigation is fundamental to grasp the components impacting everything.

At its center, smoking as a pressure help and unwinding device is established in the pharmacological impacts of nicotine, a psychoactive substance tracked down in tobacco. Nicotine's capacity to regulate synapses, especially dopamine, serotonin, and norepinephrine, adds to the prompt feeling of unwinding and mind-set height experienced by smokers. The perplexing interchange among nicotine and these synapses makes an impermanent getaway from stress, making smoking a convincing self-mitigating instrument.

The connection between stress alleviation and smoking is profoundly imbued in the physiological reactions to push. At the point when people experience stressors, the body initiates the thoughtful sensory system, setting off the arrival of stress chemicals like cortisol and adrenaline. The quieting impacts of nicotine, through its activity on synapses, go about as an offset to the physiological excitement instigated by pressure. This prompt help makes a building up circle, where people partner smoking with unwinding and stress moderation.

Mentally, smoking turns into a ritualized reaction to stretch, giving a natural and apparently powerful survival strategy. The demonstration of lighting a cigarette, enjoying conscious drags, and breathing out smoke can act as an organized and deliberate movement that diverts people from stressors. The formal idea of smoking makes a personal conduct standard that is profoundly imbued in the singular's reaction to push, adding to the apparent viability of smoking as a pressure help device.

The mental part of smoking as a pressure help system is likewise connected to molded reactions. After some time, people foster relationship among smoking and stress decrease. These learned affiliations become strong triggers, provoking people to go after a cigarette because of stress signals. The molded reaction further cements the association among smoking and stress help, forming smoking ways of behaving as a routine response to stressors.

Social and social elements assume a huge part in molding the view of smoking as a pressure help and unwinding device. The depiction of smoking in media and mainstream society frequently portrays characters going to cigarettes during snapshots of pressure or stress. These social portrayals add to the story that smoking is a feasible methodology for adapting to life's difficulties. The standardization of smoking as a pressure help device in cultural stories supports the social content, impacting people's discernments and ways of behaving.

The sociocultural setting likewise influences the accessibility and social worthiness of smoking as a pressure help system. The presence of assigned smoking regions in working environments, public spaces, and social settings can establish conditions where smoking is seen as an endorsed method for stress help. The mutual part of smoking, especially in group environments, supports that smoking isn't just a singular survival technique yet additionally a common action that encourages social associations.

The job of pressure help and unwinding in smoking way of behaving isn't uniform across all people. Varieties in pressure reaction, survival strategies, and individual contrasts add to the different ways individuals draw in with smoking as a pressure help device. A few people might find help through the quieting impacts of nicotine, while others might go to elective survival techniques like activity, care, or social help. Understanding this inconstancy is significant for fitting powerful smoking suspension mediations that address the particular necessities of people.

The fleeting part of pressure alleviation through smoking adds one more layer to the intricacy of this relationship. While smoking might give quick help from intense pressure, the drawn out influence on constant pressure is less clear. The repeating idea of stress and smoking, where smoking gives transitory help however may add to expanded pressure over the long haul, highlights the requirement for a comprehensive comprehension of the pressure smoking association.

Also, stress alleviation through smoking isn't restricted to the physiological impacts of nicotine; it stretches out to the tangible and conduct parts of the smoking experience. The material vibes of holding a cigarette, the cadenced inward breaths, and the demonstration of breathing out smoke make a multisensory experience that draws in people on an instinctive level. The tangible commitment becomes interlaced with the pressure help, adding to the in general apparent viability of smoking as an unwinding device.

Looking at the job of pressure alleviation and unwinding in smoking way of behaving likewise requires thought of co-happening emotional well-being conditions. People with nervousness, gloom, or other mind-set issues might be more defenseless to involving smoking as a survival technique for stress.

Oneself sedating theory proposes that people with psychological wellness conditions might go to smoking to mitigate side effects and direct their close to home states. Tending to the entwined connection between psychological well-being and smoking is fundamental for creating extensive intercessions.

The intricacies of stress help, unwinding, and smoking way of behaving reach out to the domain of smoking suspension. People endeavoring to stop smoking frequently face difficulties connected with the withdrawal of nicotine, the interruption of adapted reactions, and the quest for elective survival strategies. Effective smoking end programs perceive the complex idea of stress alleviation and unwinding in smoking ways of behaving, offering fitted techniques to address both the physiological and mental parts.

Understanding the job of pressure help and unwinding in smoking way of behaving is additionally essential for forestalling smoking commencement among youth. Teenagers, confronted with the difficulties of pre-adulthood and companion pressures, might be attracted to smoking for of fitting in, overseeing pressure, or opposing cultural standards. Counteraction endeavors should consider the social and social aspects that add to the allure of smoking as a pressure help device among youthful people.

General wellbeing efforts and intercessions pointed toward lessening smoking pervasiveness ought to integrate systems that challenge the story of smoking as a successful pressure help component. Advancing elective pressure the board procedures, bringing issues to light about the drawn out wellbeing results of smoking, and exposing fantasies encompassing the pressure letting properties free from cigarettes are fundamental parts of complete enemy of smoking drives.

All in all, the job of pressure help and unwinding in smoking way of behaving is a complicated transaction of physiological, mental, and sociocultural variables. The quick alleviation given by nicotine, the ritualized idea of smoking, and the molded reactions add to the impression of smoking as a compelling survival technique for stress. Social and social factors further shape the story around smoking, building up its job as a common action and a socially endorsed method for stress help.

The complexities of stress help and unwinding in smoking conduct feature the requirement for all encompassing ways to deal with smoking suspension and counteraction. Perceiving the fluctuation in individual reactions, taking into account co-happening psychological well-being conditions, and tending to the social and social elements of smoking are fundamental for creating viable mediations. Eventually, disentangling the intricacies of stress help and unwinding in smoking way of behaving is urgent for propelling comprehension we might interpret smoking as a multi-layered conduct with extensive ramifications for general wellbeing.

The interlacing of unwinding and smoking conduct frames a mind boggling embroidery that rises above simple propensity, digging into mental, physiological, and cultural aspects. Understanding the job of unwinding in smoking way of behaving requires a nuanced investigation of the variables that add to the apparent unwinding advantages of smoking, the physiological impacts of nicotine, and the sociocultural setting wherein smoking happens.

At the core of the connection among unwinding and smoking falsehoods the pharmacological effect of nicotine, the essential psychoactive substance in tobacco. Nicotine's capacity to tweak synapses, including dopamine, serotonin, and norepinephrine, makes a fountain of impacts that add to a feeling of unwinding and state of mind upgrade. The quick effect of nicotine on these synapses furnishes smokers with a brief getaway from stress, supporting the relationship among smoking and unwinding.

Physiologically, smoking prompts a complicated transaction of reactions in the body, impacting pulse, circulatory strain, and generally excitement levels. The demonstration of breathing in and breathing out smoke turns into a cadenced cycle that, for some smokers, prompts a condition of serenity. This physiological reaction adds to the apparent unwinding advantages of smoking, making a criticism circle where people partner smoking with a decrease in pressure and strain.

Mentally, smoking turns into a ritualized reaction to push, making an organized and deliberate movement that occupies people from stressors. The demonstration of lighting a cigarette, enjoying conscious drags, and breathing out smoke gives an engaged and intentional way of behaving that can immediately move consideration away from stressors. The formal idea of smoking, joined with the tactile parts of the experience, adds to the mental relationship among smoking and unwinding.

The molded reactions created after some time assume an essential part in supporting the connection among unwinding and smoking. People figure out how to connect the demonstration of smoking with pressure help, making a learned way of behaving that turns out to be profoundly instilled. The adapted reaction to push prompts further cements the association among smoking and unwinding, forming smoking ways of behaving as a programmed reaction to stressors.

Sociocultural elements contribute fundamentally to the view of smoking as an unwinding instrument. Social portrayals in media frequently portray characters going to cigarettes in snapshots of pressure, building up the account that smoking is a compelling pressure the board technique. The standardization of smoking in group environments, whether in motion pictures, TV programs, or genuine circumstances, further adds to the social content that partners smoking with unwinding and stress alleviation.

The job of unwinding in smoking way of behaving isn't uniform across all people. Varieties in pressure reaction, survival strategies, and individual contrasts add to different ways individuals draw in with smoking as an unwinding device.

While certain people might find help through the quieting impacts of nicotine, others might go to elective survival techniques like activity, care, or social help. Perceiving this fluctuation is essential for fitting smoking end mediations that address the particular necessities of people.

The tangible and social parts of smoking add to the by and large saw viability of smoking as an unwinding device. The material impressions of holding a cigarette, the musical inward breaths, and the demonstration of breathing out smoke make a multisensory experience that draws in people on an instinctive level. The tactile commitment becomes interwoven with the pressure alleviation, adding to the general unwinding benefits related with smoking.

Besides, the worldly part of unwinding through smoking adds one more layer to the intricacy of this relationship. While smoking might give quick help from intense pressure, the drawn out influence on constant pressure is less clear. The repetitive idea of stress and smoking, where smoking gives fleeting help however may add to expanded pressure over the long haul, highlights the requirement for a thorough comprehension of the unwinding smoking association.

Besides, the job of unwinding in smoking way of behaving stretches out to smoking discontinuance endeavors. People endeavoring to stop smoking frequently face difficulties connected with the withdrawal of nicotine, the disturbance of adapted reactions, and the quest for elective survival strategies. Fruitful smoking discontinuance programs perceive the complex idea of unwinding in smoking ways of behaving, offering fitted techniques to address both the physiological and mental parts.

Understanding the job of unwinding in smoking way of behaving is essential for general wellbeing efforts and mediations pointed toward decreasing smoking commonness. Advancing elective pressure the executives methods, bringing issues to light about the drawn out wellbeing results of smoking, and exposing fantasies encompassing the unwinding advantages of cigarettes are fundamental parts of thorough enemy of smoking drives.

The intricacies of unwinding and smoking way of behaving reach out to the domain of smoking inception among youth. Young people, confronted with the difficulties of pre-adulthood and companion pressures, might be attracted to smoking for the purpose of fitting in, overseeing pressure, or opposing cultural standards. Counteraction endeavors should consider the social and social aspects that add to the allure of smoking as an unwinding device among youthful people.

All in all, the job of unwinding in smoking way of behaving is a diverse transaction of physiological, mental, and sociocultural elements. The pharmacological impacts of nicotine, the physiological reactions instigated by smoking, and the mental and molded reactions add to the apparent unwinding advantages of smoking. Sociocultural factors further shape the story around smoking, supporting its job as a common movement and a socially endorsed method for unwinding.

Understanding the complexities of unwinding and smoking way of behaving is fundamental for creating compelling smoking discontinuance and counteraction systems. Perceiving the fluctuation in individual reactions, taking into account co-happening psychological well-being conditions, and tending to the social and social elements of smoking are basic for planning mediations that reverberate with different populaces. At last, unwinding the intricacies of unwinding and smoking way of behaving is pivotal for propelling comprehension we might interpret smoking as an intricate way of behaving with broad ramifications for general wellbeing.

# Chapter 8

### Smoke Signals – Global Perspectives

Smoke signals have been utilized for a really long time as a type of correspondence among different societies all over the planet. By and large, native people groups utilized smoke signals for of sending messages across immense distances, frequently in regions where different types of correspondence were illogical. The utilization of smoke signals was not restricted to a solitary district or local area; rather, it tracked down articulation in various structures across different social orders. Past its verifiable roots, the idea of smoke signals takes on new aspects in the cutting edge period, offering a figurative focal point through which to look at worldwide viewpoints on correspondence, cooperation, and the interconnectedness of our reality.

In the 21st hundred years, our method for correspondence have developed emphatically, moved by mechanical headways that have associated individuals across mainlands in a moment. The web, virtual entertainment, and cell phones have turned into the contemporary counterparts of smoke signals, filling in as conductors for the trading of data, thoughts, and culture on a worldwide scale. However, in spite of these headways, the allegorical smoke signs of our interconnected world likewise convey reverberations of difficulties and intricacies that request our consideration.

One critical part of contemporary worldwide correspondence is the effect of innovation on social trade. While the computerized age has worked with exceptional network, it has likewise brought up issues about the protection of social variety. The fast dispersal of data can prompt the homogenization of societies, as predominant stories and patterns pervade social orders around the world. In this specific situation, the figurative smoke signals become signs of social trade, where the subtleties of assorted customs risk being lost in the hurricane of globalized correspondence.

The topic of social safeguarding meets with more extensive issues of force elements and portrayal. In the worldwide correspondence scene, certain voices might be enhanced while others are minimized, making awkward nature that shape the accounts we experience. The figurative smoke signals, in this unique circumstance, become an impression of the power structures that impact the progression of data and the voices that are heard or quieted.

Besides, the worldwide idea of correspondence likewise uncovers the difficulties of exploring a world interconnected by computerized strings. The straightforwardness with which data traversed borders has significant ramifications for issues like deception, disinformation, and the spread of publicity. In the scene of figurative smoke signals, recognizing signs of truth and misrepresentation turns into a basic errand, one that requires media proficiency, decisive reasoning, and a nuanced comprehension of the perplexing snare of worldwide correspondence.

The interconnectedness of our reality isn't just obvious in that frame of mind of data trade yet additionally in the monetary, political, and ecological circles. Financial choices in a single region of the planet can send swells across mainlands, influencing vocations and forming the worldwide monetary scene. Political occasions in a single district can set off reactions and repercussions that resound universally. The allegorical smoke signals, in this specific situation, become marks of the association that describes our advanced world.

Ecological difficulties, as well, highlight the worldwide idea of our interconnectedness. Environmental change, deforestation, and contamination are issues that rise above public lines, requesting cooperative endeavors on a worldwide scale. The figurative smoke signals here take on an alternate significance, implying a call for aggregate activity to address shared difficulties that influence the prosperity of the planet and its occupants.

Amidst these difficulties, the potential for positive change additionally arises. The figurative smoke signals become encouraging signs, flagging open doors for joint effort, exchange, and aggregate critical thinking. Worldwide drives pointed toward resolving issues like destitution, imbalance, and denials of basic freedoms epitomize the force of interconnected correspondence to prepare assets, encourage understanding, and drive positive change on a worldwide scale.

The job of people in forming the account of worldwide interconnectedness couldn't possibly be more significant. In reality as we know it where each individual can add to the progression of data, the allegorical smoke signals become channels through which individual stories, points of view, and encounters are shared. Web-based entertainment stages, web journals, and online gatherings act as spaces where people can enhance their voices and interface with other people who might be universes away. This democratization of correspondence enables people to be dynamic members in forming the accounts that characterize our globalized world.

Nonetheless, the democratization of correspondence likewise brings difficulties connected with the veracity of data and the potential for the enhancement of destructive stories. The figurative smoke signals, when misshaped or controlled, can become devices of falsehood that spread trepidation, division, and doubt. Exploring this scene requires a guarantee to media education, moral correspondence, and an acknowledgment of the obligation that accompanies the ability to shape stories on a worldwide scale.

In investigating worldwide points of view on smoke signals, recognizing the job of language as a crucial part of communication is fundamental. The variety of dialects spoken all over the planet mirrors the extravagance of human culture and thought. Be that as it may, the globalized idea of correspondence has additionally prompted the strength of specific dialects in web-based spaces and worldwide talk. The figurative smoke signals, in this specific circumstance, become semantic images that convey with them the power elements of language, molding who is heard, comprehended, and addressed in the worldwide discussion.

Language fills in as a device for correspondence as well as a storehouse of social information and character. The figurative smoke signals, when grounded in etymological variety, become a festival of the horde manners by which human social orders express their encounters, values, and desires. Endeavors to advance phonetic variety in the computerized age are fundamental for saving the wealth of human articulation and guaranteeing that no voice is lost or minimized in the huge ocean of worldwide correspondence.

In the domain of worldwide viewpoints, the figurative smoke signals reach out to the domain of strategy and global relations. Countries speak with each other through conciliatory channels, settlements, and worldwide associations, making a complicated snare of connections that shape the international scene. The figurative smoke signals here become emblematic motions, strategy choices, and international moves that impact the course of history and characterize the connections between countries on the worldwide stage.

The difficulties looked by the worldwide local area, from clashes and philanthropic emergencies to general wellbeing crises, highlight the requirement for powerful worldwide correspondence and participation.

The figurative smoke signals, in this unique circumstance, become pressing calls for joint effort, compassion, and fortitude even with shared difficulties that rise above public limits. The interconnected idea of our reality requests an aggregate reaction that perceives the relationship of countries and the common obligation to resolve worldwide issues.

In looking at worldwide points of view on smoke signals, it is essential to consider the job of innovation as both an empowering agent and a disruptor of correspondence. The advanced age has achieved remarkable open doors for association, permitting individuals from various corners of the world to take part continuously correspondence, coordinated effort, and social trade. The allegorical smoke signals, in this mechanically determined time, become the zeros and ones of computerized code that navigate the tremendous organization of the web, associating people and networks in manners unbelievable in past periods.

However, the very innovation that works with worldwide correspondence likewise presents difficulties to protection, security, and moral contemplations. The allegorical smoke signals, when sent through computerized channels, bring up issues about information assurance, observation, and the potential for maltreatment of innovative power. As we explore the intricacies of the computerized scene, it becomes vital for find some kind of harmony between bridling the advantages of innovation and defending the rules that support moral and mindful correspondence in a globalized world.

The effect of innovation on correspondence is additionally highlighted by the ascent of man-made reasoning and robotization. The figurative smoke signals, in this specific situation, take on a cutting edge aspect, representing the calculations, AI, and mechanized frameworks that shape the data we experience on the web. The ramifications of computer based intelligence for the fate of work, navigation, and human collaboration are significant, provoking reflections on the moral contemplations and cultural ramifications of a reality where machines assume an undeniably focal part in molding the stories of our interconnected presence.

The figurative smoke signs of our globalized world additionally stretch out to the domain of social and social developments. The force of aggregate activity, intensified through computerized stages, has brought about developments that rise above public boundaries and point out issues like civil rights, ecological maintainability, and common liberties. The figurative smoke signals, in this unique circumstance, become the revitalizing cries, hashtags, and viral missions that prepare people and networks to advocate for positive change on a worldwide scale.

Be that as it may, the worldwide idea of these developments additionally features the difficulties of making an interpretation of online activism into unmistakable, true effect. The allegorical smoke signals, when restricted to the computerized domain, may battle to impact foundational change without disconnected commitment, grassroots getting sorted out, and supported endeavors to address the underlying drivers of the main things.

Exploring the convergence of online activism and on-the-ground influence requires a nuanced comprehension of the elements of social change in a globalized setting.

In investigating worldwide points of view on smoke signals, it is fundamental to perceive the job of schooling in molding how people draw in with and add to the worldwide discussion. The figurative smoke signals, when grounded in schooling, become images of information, decisive reasoning, and social mindfulness. In an interconnected world, schooling turns into a useful asset for cultivating a worldwide outlook that rises above social limits and advances a profound comprehension of the intricacies that characterize our common presence.

Worldwide training likewise assumes a pivotal part in tending to the computerized partition, guaranteeing that people all over the planet approach the devices and abilities expected to explore the advanced scene. The allegorical smoke signals, in this unique situation, become guides of admittance to data, advanced education, and potential open doors for people to take part genuinely in the worldwide discussion. Spanning the computerized partition isn't just an issue of innovative framework yet in addition of impartial admittance to schooling that engages people to explore the intricacies of our interconnected world.

As we consider worldwide viewpoints on smoke signals, it becomes apparent that the illustration reaches out past the advanced domain to incorporate the more extensive subject of human association and reliance. The figurative smoke signals become images of the strings that tight spot us all together local area, rising above lines, societies, and contrasts. In our current reality where the difficulties we face are progressively interconnected, the figurative smoke signals call for cooperation, understanding, and a common obligation to building an all the more, reasonable, and comprehensive future.

### 8.1 International variations in smoking prevalence

Global varieties in smoking pervasiveness offer a nuanced focal point through which to look at the complicated exchange of social, financial, and general wellbeing factors that shape tobacco use all over the planet. Smoking, a conduct well established in history and cultural standards, has turned into a worldwide wellbeing worry with huge ramifications for individual prosperity and general wellbeing frameworks. Examining the pervasiveness of smoking on a worldwide scale uncovers examples, abberations, and difficulties that highlight the requirement for extensive methodologies to address this worldwide medical problem.

Understanding the varieties in smoking commonness requires a thought of the verifiable, social, and monetary settings that impact tobacco use in various locales. The foundations of smoking can be followed back hundreds of years, with tobacco assuming a part in ceremonies, social communications, and exchange among native networks some time before the appearance of Europeans in the Americas. The social meaning of tobacco changed broadly, from consecrated functions to restorative works on, mirroring the variety of viewpoints on this plant.

Notwithstanding, the worldwide spread of tobacco use took an extraordinary turn with the appearance of European wayfarers in the fifteenth and sixteenth hundreds of years. The development and commercialization of tobacco became interlaced with colonization and exchange, prompting the broad utilization of tobacco items around the world. The authentic setting established the groundwork for the assorted social mentalities towards smoking that continue right up to the present day, molding the commonness of smoking in various social orders.

Social elements assume a vital part in molding smoking ways of behaving, as normal practices, customs, and impression of tobacco impact whether smoking is acknowledged or derided inside a local area. In certain societies, smoking is profoundly imbued in friendly customs and is viewed as a soul changing experience or an image of adulthood. Then again, in different social orders, smoking might be disapproved of, related with wellbeing dangers, and dependent upon general wellbeing efforts putting its utilization down.

The social meaning of smoking stretches out past individual ways of behaving to more extensive cultural perspectives and strategies. In certain nations, smoking might be profoundly implanted in social practices, with tobacco filling in as an image of cordiality or social association. Understanding these social subtleties is critical for planning successful tobacco control estimates that regard social variety and draw in with networks in a significant way.

Monetary factors likewise contribute altogether to worldwide varieties in smoking predominance. The tobacco business, a worldwide monetary force to be reckoned with, assumes a focal part in molding examples of tobacco use. In certain locales, tobacco development fills in as an imperative monetary action, giving jobs to ranchers and adding to the financial improvement of whole networks. The monetary interests attached to tobacco creation can make difficulties for executing hostile to smoking strategies, as states might be hesitant to risk a worthwhile industry.

In addition, the globalized idea of the tobacco business permits worldwide enterprises to showcase and disperse tobacco items across borders, affecting smoking examples in different social and monetary settings. Forceful showcasing techniques, frequently focusing on weak populaces, add to the propagation of smoking in specific districts. The financial interests of the tobacco business in this way meet with social standards, making a mind boggling scene that requires complex ways to deal with address smoking pervasiveness.

General wellbeing drives pointed toward diminishing smoking predominance should explore this complex trap of social and financial elements to be compelling. Worldwide endeavors, for example, the Structure Show on Tobacco Control (FCTC) created by the World Wellbeing Association (WHO), look to give a planned and complete reaction to the worldwide tobacco scourge. The FCTC stresses proof based systems, including tobacco tax collection, publicizing limitations, and backing for smoking end programs, to address the diverse difficulties presented by tobacco use.

In spite of these worldwide endeavors, huge varieties in smoking commonness endure, featuring the requirement for setting explicit mediations customized to the exceptional difficulties looked by every locale. In big league salary nations, where tobacco control measures are more common and public familiarity with smoking dangers is for the most part higher, smoking predominance will in general be lower. In any case, in low-and center pay nations, where assets for general wellbeing efforts might be restricted, and tobacco control strategies less severe, smoking pervasiveness stays a squeezing concern.

One element adding to the tirelessness of smoking in specific districts is the commonness of smoking among explicit segment gatherings. For instance, orientation assumes a critical part in smoking examples, with varieties saw among people in various regions of the planet. In certain social orders, smoking might be all the more socially OK for men, prompting higher smoking rates among guys. Then again, in different societies, smoking among ladies might be dependent upon more prominent shame, bringing about lower generally speaking smoking pervasiveness yet possibly higher rates among explicit segment gatherings.

Age is another basic segment factor impacting smoking commonness.

Commencement into smoking frequently happens during youthfulness, and the variables affecting this inception fluctuate broadly across locales. Peer pressure, openness to tobacco showcasing, and financial factors all add to the take-up of smoking among youngsters. Understanding the elements of smoking inception among various age bunches is fundamental for planning designated avoidance techniques that address the special difficulties looked by youths and youthful grown-ups.

The effect of smoking stretches out past individual wellbeing to more extensive general wellbeing contemplations. The relationship among smoking and a scope of medical problems, including respiratory sicknesses, cardiovascular illnesses, and different types of disease, highlights the criticalness of tending to smoking predominance as a general wellbeing need. In districts where smoking rates are high, the weight on medical services frameworks can be significant, with expanded medical care expenses and burden on assets.

The variations in smoking pervasiveness additionally add to worldwide wellbeing imbalances, both inside and between nations. Financial variables, including pay and training levels, frequently converge with smoking examples, with higher smoking rates saw among minimized and hindered populaces. The test of tending to smoking as a general medical problem requires a thorough methodology that thinks about the social determinants of wellbeing, recognizing the interconnected idea of elements that add to smoking pervasiveness.

Smoking discontinuance projects and arrangements are indispensable parts of endeavors to decrease smoking pervasiveness all around the world. Notwithstanding, the viability of these mediations can shift in light of social, monetary, and social elements.

Fitting smoking suspension drives to the particular requirements and inclinations of different populaces is pivotal for advancing fruitful results. This might include considering social standards around wellbeing looking for ways of behaving, planning efforts that resound with neighborhood networks, and giving open assets to people hoping to stop smoking.

In certain locales, where smoking is profoundly dug in social practices, hurt decrease methodologies may likewise assume a part in tending to smoking-related wellbeing gambles. Hurt decrease approaches mean to limit the unfortunate results of tobacco use without fundamentally pushing for complete restraint. This could include advancing the utilization of less destructive tobacco items, like electronic cigarettes, as an option in contrast to conventional smoking. In any case, the viability and moral contemplations of mischief decrease procedures remain subjects of discussion inside the general wellbeing local area.

The job of government approaches in forming smoking commonness couldn't possibly be more significant. Tobacco control measures, including tax assessment, publicizing limitations, and without smoke strategies, have shown adequacy in diminishing smoking rates in numerous nations. Notwithstanding, the political will to carry out and implement such arrangements fluctuates, and the impact of the tobacco business on policymaking can introduce critical snags.

Tax collection, specifically, has demonstrated to be an incredible asset in decreasing smoking pervasiveness. Higher tobacco costs have been related with diminished smoking rates, particularly among weak populaces, like youth and low-pay people. Furthermore, publicizing limitations limit the business' capacity to showcase and advance tobacco items, decreasing the allure of smoking, especially among more youthful socioeconomics.

Sans smoke arrangements, which limit smoking in broad daylight spaces, working environments, and other shared conditions, add to switching cultural standards up smoking. These arrangements shield non-smokers from handed-down cigarette smoke as well as add to denormalizing smoking, supporting the message that smoking is unsafe and socially unsatisfactory.

While some big time salary nations have effectively executed vigorous tobacco control gauges, the difficulties in low-and center pay nations highlight the requirement for worldwide fortitude in tending to smoking pervasiveness. Worldwide joint efforts, asset sharing, and information trade can assume a pivotal part in supporting nations with less assets in their endeavors to carry out successful tobacco control strategies.

## 8.2 Government policies and anti-smoking initiatives around the world

Government strategies and hostile to smoking drives all over the planet address a basic reaction to the worldwide wellbeing challenge presented by smoking. Tobacco use stays a main source of preventable demise and infection, inciting legislatures to execute a scope of measures to control smoking commonness, safeguard general wellbeing, and moderate the monetary and social weights related with tobacco-related diseases. Inspecting the different methodologies utilized by states offers bits of knowledge into the intricacies of hostile to smoking endeavors, the effect of social and monetary variables, and the developing scene of tobacco control on a worldwide scale.

One foundation of government endeavors to battle smoking is the execution of tobacco tax collection arrangements. Tax collection fills in as an integral asset to prevent smoking by expanding the expense of tobacco items. Greater costs make cigarettes more expensive, especially for cost touchy socioeconomics like youth and low-pay people. Various examinations have shown a reasonable relationship between's expanded tobacco burdens and decreased smoking rates, adding to the general decrease in tobacco use in numerous nations.

Nonetheless, the adequacy of tobacco tax assessment relies upon a few variables, including the size of the expense increment, the presence of illegal tobacco markets, and the financial setting of the populace. States should figure out some kind of harmony between raising costs to deter smoking and keeping away from potentially negative side-effects, for example, the development of unlawful tobacco exchange or lopsided financial weights on specific gatherings.

Notwithstanding tax collection, publicizing limitations assume a urgent part in molding the tobacco control scene. State run administrations all over the planet have executed measures to restrict the showcasing and advancement of tobacco items, perceiving the job of publicizing in empowering smoking commencement and supporting tobacco enslavement. Thorough prohibitions on tobacco publicizing, advancement, and sponsorship add to switching cultural standards up smoking, decreasing the perceivability and allure of tobacco items.

The viability of publicizing limitations is additionally intensified by endeavors to execute realistic wellbeing admonitions on cigarette bundling. Realistic alerts utilize visual pictures to portray the wellbeing outcomes of smoking, planning to impart the dangers in a more effective manner than printed admonitions alone. The blend of publicizing limitations and realistic wellbeing admonitions fills in as a strong hindrance, particularly among youth and possible new smokers.

Sans smoke strategies address one more key component of against smoking drives, safeguarding the two smokers and non-smokers from the unsafe impacts of handed-down cigarette smoke.

State run administrations overall have executed regulations and guidelines to limit smoking in broad daylight spaces, working environments, and cordiality scenes. These strategies add to the denormalization of smoking, supporting the message that smoking isn't just an individual wellbeing risk yet in addition a general wellbeing concern.

The progress of without smoke arrangements is dependent upon compelling execution and implementation. Hearty arrangements joined with public mindfulness crusades assist with moving normal practices and diminish the social adequacy of smoking in shared spaces. Be that as it may, difficulties might emerge in areas where social standards or financial interests struggle with the severe requirement of sans smoke strategies.

Correlative to these administrative measures, smoking discontinuance programs are instrumental in supporting people in their endeavors to stop smoking. Government-supported drives, frequently conveyed through medical care frameworks, give assets, guiding, and in some cases pharmacological mediations to help smokers in their quit endeavors. Perceiving the habit-forming nature of nicotine, these projects mean to address both the physical and mental parts of tobacco reliance.

Admittance to smoking discontinuance administrations fluctuates worldwide, with big time salary nations by and large having more far reaching and available projects. Conversely, low-and center pay nations might confront difficulties in asset portion and framework for conveying viable suspension support. Overcoming this issue is pivotal for guaranteeing that people overall approach the instruments and backing they need to defeat tobacco fixation.

Hostile to smoking drives likewise reach out to the domain of government funded schooling efforts, which assume a fundamental part in bringing issues to light about the wellbeing dangers of smoking and advancing conduct change. States influence different correspondence stations, including TV, radio, print media, and computerized stages, to disperse against smoking messages. The viability of these missions depends on their capacity to reverberate with different crowds, considering social, etymological, and financial elements.

Past customary media, the ascent of computerized stages and online entertainment has set out new open doors and difficulties for hostile to smoking correspondence. State run administrations and general wellbeing associations use online channels to arrive at more youthful socioeconomics, where smoking commencement frequently happens. Nonetheless, the computerized scene additionally presents difficulties, as tobacco organizations influence virtual entertainment for designated showcasing, possibly subverting against smoking endeavors.

Worldwide coordinated efforts and arrangements further shape the scene of government strategies on smoking.

The Structure Show on Tobacco Control (FCTC), created by the World Wellbeing Association (WHO), addresses a worldwide work to address the transnational idea of the tobacco scourge. Taken on in 2003, the FCTC gives a thorough system to tobacco control, underscoring proof based procedures, worldwide collaboration, and strategy coordination.

The FCTC frames a scope of measures, including those connected with tax collection, promoting, sans smoke strategies, and bundling alerts, planning to direct nations in creating and carrying out compelling tobacco control arrangements. Starting around my last information update in January 2022, north of 180 nations are gatherings to the FCTC, mirroring a worldwide obligation to aggregate activity against the tobacco pandemic.

Nonetheless, challenges continue guaranteeing the full execution of FCTC proposals. Tobacco industry impedance, legitimate debates, and the developing scene of tobacco items, for example, e-cigarettes, present continuous difficulties for state run administrations and general wellbeing advocates. The requirement for proceeded with worldwide participation stays vital to address the advancing strategies of the tobacco business and advance successful tobacco control systems internationally.

Social factors essentially impact the outcome of government strategies and hostile to smoking drives. Social standards around smoking, impression of tobacco use, and verifiable associations with tobacco all shape the receptivity of populaces to hostile to smoking measures. In certain societies, smoking might be profoundly implanted in friendly practices, ceremonies, or soul changing experiences, presenting difficulties for mediations that plan to move these social standards.

Tobacco organizations frequently exploit social settings to showcase their items, partner smoking with thoughts of autonomy, disobedience, or refinement. States trying to balance these impacts should explore social responsive qualities, fitting enemy of smoking efforts to reverberate with nearby qualities and customs. A nuanced comprehension of social elements is fundamental to guarantee that mediations are socially able and conscious of different viewpoints.

Monetary contemplations additionally influence the progress of against smoking drives. In districts where tobacco development is a critical financial movement, endeavors to diminish smoking might confront opposition from partners dependent on the tobacco business. Legislatures should explore the fragile harmony between general wellbeing goals and the monetary interests of tobacco ranchers and industry laborers. Executing systems for financial enhancement in tobacco-subordinate locales becomes vital to guarantee a simply change away from tobacco development.

The moderateness and openness of tobacco items likewise impact smoking pervasiveness. In some low-and center pay nations, where dispensable earnings are lower, the moderately lower cost of tobacco items can add to higher smoking rates. Tobacco tax collection fills in as an immediate system to resolve this issue, making cigarettes more expensive and consequently decreasing utilization, particularly among cost delicate populaces.

The developing scene of tobacco items represents extra difficulties for government arrangements and hostile to smoking drives. The development of e-cigarettes and other novel tobacco and nicotine conveyance frameworks presents new contemplations for guideline and general wellbeing. While some view e-cigarettes as a possibly less destructive option in contrast to conventional smoking, concerns exist about their drawn out wellbeing impacts, particularly among youth.

Legislatures wrestle with finding some kind of harmony between permitting grown-up smokers admittance to possibly less unsafe choices while forestalling the inception of tobacco use, especially among youngsters. Administrative structures for e-cigarettes differ worldwide, for certain nations embracing hurt decrease techniques and others taking on a prudent methodology.

Government approaches and hostile to smoking drives should likewise address wellbeing differences inside populaces. Smoking predominance frequently changes in light of financial elements, with higher rates saw among minimized and impeded networks. Fitting intercessions to address these variations requires a complex methodology that thinks about the social determinants of wellbeing, including pay, training, and admittance to medical services.

### 8.3 Cultural attitudes towards smoking in different societies

Social mentalities towards smoking change broadly across various social orders, mirroring a complicated interaction of verifiable, social, and financial variables that shape view of tobacco use. Smoking has profound authentic roots, and its social importance has advanced over the long run, adding to assorted perspectives and practices all over the planet. Looking at these social subtleties gives bits of knowledge into the difficulties and open doors for tobacco control endeavors and features the significance of setting explicit ways to deal with address smoking predominance.

All things considered, smoking has held assorted social implications, going from sacrosanct ceremonies to social traditions. In a few native societies, tobacco assumed a focal part in otherworldly services, representing correspondence with the heavenly or associating with predecessors. The sacrosanct utilization of tobacco was frequently particular from the sporting or habit-forming utilize that arose later with the spread of tobacco through worldwide exchange.

The acquaintance of tobacco with various areas of the planet by European pilgrims in the fifteenth and sixteenth hundreds of years changed its social importance. Tobacco became laced with exchange, colonization, and cultural practices. In certain societies, smoking was embraced as an image of refinement or recreation, while in others, it took on formal or restorative jobs. The verifiable setting of tobacco's presentation and reception molded the establishment for different social perspectives towards smoking.

Social mentalities towards smoking frequently cross with more extensive cultural standards, including impression of orientation jobs. In certain social orders, smoking is profoundly gendered, with explicit assumptions or restrictions around smoking for people. Gendered social standards might impact the predominance of smoking among various sexes and effect how smoking is seen inside networks.

For instance, in specific societies, smoking among men might be viewed as a transitional experience, a marker of adulthood, or an image of manliness. Conversely, smoking among ladies could convey various implications, possibly confronting more prominent shame because of cultural assumptions or impression of gentility. These gendered social standards add to varieties in smoking pervasiveness and examples across various social orders.

Strict convictions likewise assume a critical part in forming social perspectives towards smoking. In certain societies, smoking is seen through a strict focal point, with rehearses established in strict ceremonies or restrictions. Certain strict practices might deter or forbid smoking, affecting the predominance of smoking inside strict networks. Alternately, in different societies, smoking might be coordinated into strict services or works on, mirroring the variety of points of view on tobacco use.

Understanding social mentalities towards smoking requires an enthusiasm for the job of tobacco in friendly communications and local area elements. Smoking is many times implanted in friendly customs, get-togethers, or common exercises, filling in as a common encounter that encourages associations among people. These social components of smoking add to its social importance, making it a mind boggling conduct entwined with social holding and personality development.

The standardization of smoking inside groups of friends can introduce difficulties for against smoking drives, as intercessions should explore dug in social practices and relational elements. Smoking discontinuance endeavors might profit from perceiving and utilizing existing social designs to advance better ways of behaving, recognizing the significance of local area commitment in molding social mentalities towards smoking.

Financial contemplations likewise impact social mentalities towards smoking, particularly in locales where tobacco development is a huge monetary action.

In people group subject to tobacco cultivating, the social meaning of tobacco might be intently attached to jobs and monetary maintainability. Endeavors to move social mentalities towards smoking in these settings should address the financial difficulties looked by networks dependent on the tobacco business, accentuating the requirement for elective monetary open doors.

The depiction of smoking in mainstream society, including motion pictures, TV, and promoting, further shapes social mentalities towards tobacco use. The media's impact on view of smoking can add to the standardization of tobacco use or, on the other hand, support against smoking messages. Social perspectives might be impacted by how smoking is portrayed in mainstream society, influencing the social worthiness of smoking inside a given society.

Government arrangements and guidelines likewise add to molding social mentalities towards smoking. Rigid tobacco control measures, including promoting limitations, realistic wellbeing admonitions, and without smoke strategies, can impact cultural standards and impression of smoking. The outcome of such arrangements relies upon their arrangement with social qualities, viable correspondence methodologies, and joint effort with networks to guarantee that mediations reverberate with nearby settings.

In certain social orders, government strategies might confront obstruction in the event that they are seen as encroaching upon social practices or individual opportunities. Offsetting general wellbeing goals with social contemplations is vital for the fruitful execution of tobacco control measures. Social skill in arrangement plan and execution includes perceiving and regarding different social perspectives towards smoking while at the same time focusing on the general objective of safeguarding general wellbeing.

The globalized idea of correspondence and the impact of Western social standards through media and promoting additionally add to the dissemination of specific perspectives towards smoking. The depiction of smoking as an image of defiance, freedom, or refinement in Western mainstream society widespreadly affects view of tobacco utilize around the world. Nearby societies may either oppose or embrace these imported social stories, further molding their own perspectives towards smoking.

The advancing scene of tobacco items, including the ascent of e-cigarettes and novel tobacco conveyance frameworks, acquaints new aspects with social perspectives towards smoking. While certain social orders might embrace hurt decrease approaches and view these options as less unsafe than conventional smoking, others might move toward them with wariness or incredulity. Social perspectives towards arising tobacco items add to the intricacies of tobacco control endeavors, requiring versatile systems to address developing examples of tobacco use.

Social perspectives towards smoking are not static; they develop after some time in light of evolving social, financial, and political elements.

The outcome of hostile to smoking drives relies on perceiving the powerful idea of social mentalities and adjusting intercessions to line up with developing cultural standards. Socially touchy methodologies that connect with networks, influence existing social designs, and regard assorted points of view are fundamental for encouraging manageable changes in social perspectives towards smoking.

All in all, social mentalities towards smoking are multi-layered and molded by a perplexing transaction of verifiable, social, monetary, and political variables. Perceiving the variety of social points of view on tobacco use is fundamental for planning compelling and socially touchy enemy of smoking drives. The crossing point of smoking with social, gendered, strict, and monetary aspects features the requirement for nuanced approaches that regard social variety while tending to the worldwide wellbeing challenge presented by smoking. As social orders keep on developing, understanding and adjusting to changing social perspectives towards smoking will stay a significant part of thorough tobacco control endeavors around the world.

Smoking in various social orders is a mind boggling and diverse peculiarity impacted by a bunch of elements, including social, social, financial, and political contemplations. The pervasiveness and mentalities towards smoking change generally across the globe, mirroring the remarkable verifiable, customary, and contemporary settings of every general public. Investigating the assorted scene of smoking in various social orders gives significant bits of knowledge into the difficulties and potential open doors for tobacco control endeavors and highlights the requirement for socially fitted ways to deal with address this worldwide medical problem.

Social mentalities towards smoking assume a focal part in forming the examples of tobacco use inside a general public. Smoking has profound verifiable roots, and its social importance has developed after some time. In certain social orders, smoking is implanted in old practices and ceremonies, frequently holding representative or strict implications. For instance, certain native societies integrate tobacco into hallowed functions, seeing it as a channel for correspondence with the profound domain or as a fundamental piece of social practices.

Be that as it may, the social meaning of smoking isn't uniform across all social orders. The acquaintance of tobacco with various regions of the planet through pilgrim shipping lanes changed its social meanings. In certain societies, smoking became related with relaxation, refinement, or economic wellbeing. In others, it kept up with formal or restorative jobs. The authentic setting of tobacco's acquaintance and reception contributed with assorted social mentalities towards smoking that persevere today.

Orientation elements essentially impact how smoking is seen inside various social orders. Social standards around orientation jobs influence the predominance and social adequacy of smoking among people. In certain societies, smoking is profoundly gendered, with explicit assumptions or restrictions around smoking for every orientation.

For example, in specific social orders, smoking among men might be seen as an indication of manliness, while smoking among ladies might be dependent upon more prominent disgrace because of cultural assumptions connected with gentility.

These gendered social standards add to varieties in smoking predominance and examples across various social orders. General wellbeing mediations tending to smoking in such settings should consider these orientation elements to foster successful techniques that reverberate with social qualities and standards.

Strict convictions likewise shape social mentalities towards smoking, as certain religions might deter or forbid tobacco use while others coordinate it into strict functions. In social orders where religion assumes a focal part, smoking might be seen through a moral or moral focal point, impacting both individual and collective impression of tobacco use. The exchange between strict lessons and social mentalities towards smoking requires nuanced approaches in tobacco control endeavors to explore the intricacies of conviction frameworks.

The depiction of smoking in mainstream society further forms social mentalities towards tobacco use. Films, TV, and promoting add to the standardization of smoking or, on the other hand, build up enemy of smoking messages. The portrayal of smoking in mainstream society can impact how smoking is seen inside a general public, influencing normal practices and worthiness. State run administrations and general wellbeing advocates frequently wrestle with the test of checking supportive of smoking impacts in famous media while advancing enemy of smoking messages that resound with different crowds.

Financial contemplations add one more layer to the social components of smoking. In districts where tobacco development is a critical financial action, social perspectives towards smoking might be intently attached to occupations and monetary maintainability. Networks reliant upon tobacco cultivating may oppose hostile to smoking drives, underscoring the requirement for complete methodologies that address monetary difficulties and give elective open doors to supportable turn of events.

Besides, the reasonableness and openness of tobacco items impact smoking commonness inside various social orders. The monetary differences between big time salary and low-pay nations add to varieties in smoking examples. In some low-pay social orders, where dispensable wages are lower, the moderately lower cost of tobacco items can add to higher smoking rates. Tobacco tax collection and financial approaches become pivotal apparatuses in tending to these differences and decreasing smoking predominance.

The impact of Western social standards through globalization and media has additionally affected social mentalities towards smoking around the world. The depiction of smoking as an image of resistance, freedom, or complexity in Western mainstream society has impacted worldwide impression of tobacco use.

Neighborhood societies may either oppose or embrace these imported social accounts, further molding their own mentalities towards smoking. The dispersion of Western social impacts highlights the interconnected idea of smoking across different social orders.

Government strategies and guidelines assume a vital part in forming social perspectives towards smoking. Rigid tobacco control measures, including tax collection, publicizing limitations, realistic wellbeing admonitions, and sans smoke strategies, add to the making of hostile to smoking standards inside a general public. The outcome of such arrangements relies upon their arrangement with social qualities, powerful correspondence systems, and joint effort with networks to guarantee that intercessions reverberate with neighborhood settings.

Notwithstanding, government approaches might confront obstruction in the event that they are seen as encroaching upon social practices or individual opportunities.

Finding some kind of harmony between general wellbeing goals and social contemplations is fundamental for the effective execution of tobacco control measures. Socially skilled strategy plan and execution include perceiving and regarding assorted social mentalities towards smoking while at the same time focusing on the all-encompassing objective of safeguarding general wellbeing.

The globalized idea of correspondence and the impact of Western social standards through media and promoting additionally add to the dissemination of specific perspectives towards smoking. The depiction of smoking as an image of disobedience, freedom, or complexity in Western mainstream society widespreadly affects impression of tobacco utilize around the world. Neighborhood societies may either oppose or take on these imported social accounts, further molding their own mentalities towards smoking.

The developing scene of tobacco items represents extra difficulties for government arrangements and against smoking drives. The development of e-cigarettes and other novel tobacco and nicotine conveyance frameworks acquaints new aspects with social perspectives towards smoking. While certain social orders might embrace hurt decrease approaches and view these options as less unsafe than conventional smoking, others might move toward them with mindfulness or suspicion. Social mentalities towards arising tobacco items add to the intricacies of tobacco control endeavors, requiring versatile procedures to address advancing examples of tobacco use.

Social mentalities towards smoking are not static; they advance over the long haul in light of evolving social, monetary, and political elements. The progress of hostile to smoking drives relies on perceiving the unique idea of social perspectives and adjusting intercessions to line up with advancing cultural standards. Socially touchy methodologies that draw in networks, influence existing social designs, and regard assorted points of view are fundamental for encouraging maintainable changes in social mentalities towards smoking.

# Chapter 9

### Clearing the Air – The Path Forward

In a time characterized by fast mechanical headways, socio-political intricacies, and worldwide interconnectedness, the need to address ecological difficulties has become more squeezing than any other time. The ghost of environmental change poses a potential threat, causing qualms about the planet's future. As social orders wrestle with the results of uncontrolled industrialization and impractical practices, the basic to eliminate any confusion and clear a feasible way ahead has never been more basic.

One of the chief difficulties confronting mankind is air contamination, an unavoidable threat that rises above topographical limits and influences the wellbeing and prosperity of millions. From clamoring cities to far off country regions, no side of the globe is invulnerable to the pernicious impacts of dirtied air. Respiratory illnesses, cardiovascular complexities, and a large group of other medical problems are on the ascent, making a general wellbeing emergency of phenomenal extents.

To fathom the weightiness of the circumstance, one should dig into the sources and signs of air contamination. The burning of petroleum products, modern discharges, vehicular exhaust, and deforestation on the whole add to the corruption of air quality. These anthropogenic exercises discharge a mixed drink of contaminations into the air, including particulate matter, nitrogen oxides, sulfur dioxide, and unpredictable natural mixtures. The combined effect of these contaminations stretches out past prompt wellbeing concerns, affecting environments, biodiversity, and the general equilibrium of the planet.

Moderating air contamination requests a complex methodology that tends to its main drivers and lays out reasonable other options. The progress to environmentally friendly power sources stands apart as a urgent move toward this bearing. Embracing sun powered, wind, hydro, and other clean energy choices can altogether diminish the dependence on petroleum derivatives, checking the emanations liable for air contamination. Legislatures, organizations, and people should team up to speed up the reception of environmentally friendly power innovations, cultivating a change in outlook toward a cleaner, more reasonable energy scene.

Moreover, reexamining transportation frameworks is central in the mission to dispel any confusion. The expansion of ignition motor vehicles has been a significant supporter of air contamination. The advancement of electric vehicles, interest in open transportation foundation, and the improvement of non-mechanized methods of driving are essential parts of a supportable transportation methodology. Strategies boosting the utilization of clean vehicles, combined with rigid outflows norms, can catalyze the change to a cleaner, more productive transportation framework.

Modern exercises, one more critical wellspring of air contamination, require a change in perspective towards greener practices. Rigid natural guidelines, combined with motivations for eco-accommodating innovations, can urge businesses to take on practical creation processes. The execution of roundabout economy standards, where waste is limited, and assets are proficiently used, can additionally alleviate the natural effect of modern tasks. Coordinated effort between states, industry partners, and ecological associations is critical to encouraging an aggregate obligation to feasible modern practices.

Couple with tending to the wellsprings of contamination, a hearty checking and implementation structure is fundamental. Legislatures should put resources into cutting edge air quality observing frameworks to follow poison levels and distinguish areas of interest. Straightforward announcing components and constant information dispersal engage networks to make informed moves to safeguard their wellbeing. At the same time, rigid requirement of natural guidelines is principal to considering polluters responsible. Punishments for rebelliousness ought to be adequately impediment, cultivating a culture of corporate obligation and natural stewardship.

Be that as it may, the fight against air contamination reaches out past administrative measures and innovative arrangements. Public mindfulness and schooling assume a crucial part in cultivating a feeling of natural obligation. Drives to instruct residents about the causes and outcomes of air contamination can affect conduct change. Local area drove endeavors, grassroots developments, and instructive missions add to a more extensive cultural shift towards supportable living. By developing a comprehension of the interconnectedness between human exercises and ecological prosperity, people become dynamic members in the aggregate undertaking to eliminate any confusion.

The job of innovation in battling air contamination couldn't possibly be more significant. Developments in air cleansing advancements, for example, high level filtration frameworks and air quality observing gadgets, offer substantial answers for alleviate the effect of contamination. Innovative work in feasible materials and assembling processes add to decreasing the natural impression of items. Also, arising advancements like carbon catch and capacity present promising roads for moderating the emanations from existing modern cycles.

Worldwide coordinated effort is basic in tending to the transboundary idea of air contamination. Nations should meet up to plan and carry out methodologies that rise above international limits. Arrangements and deals that set worldwide norms for discharges, deforestation, and manageable improvement can give a structure to aggregate activity. By cultivating a feeling of coordinated effort, the global local area can pool assets, share information, and by and large work towards a cleaner, better planet.

The job of organizations in the excursion towards cleaner air couldn't possibly be more significant. Corporate manageability drives, dependable store network the board, and adherence to moral strategic policies add to decreasing the ecological effect of business exercises. Customers, outfitted with data about organizations' natural practices, can settle on scrupulous decisions, leaning toward organizations focused on manageable and eco-accommodating practices. The coordination of natural, social, and administration (ESG) measures in speculation choices further boosts organizations to focus on manageability.

Chasing cleaner air, the conservation and rebuilding of biological systems arise as indispensable parts. Woods, wetlands, and other normal territories go about as carbon sinks, retaining toxins and relieving the effect of human exercises on air quality. Preservation endeavors, afforestation projects, and the insurance of biodiversity add to making a strong environment that can more readily endure the tensions of industrialization. Perceiving the characteristic worth of nature and integrating it into metropolitan preparation and improvement is fundamental for making supportable, decent spaces.

Training and exploration are mainstays of progress in the mission for cleaner air. Putting resources into research drives that investigate imaginative answers for air contamination, environmental change, and ecological debasement is basic.

Scholastic foundations, research focuses, and think tanks assume a critical part in producing information that illuminates strategy choices and mechanical headways. By supporting a culture of logical request and scholarly interest, social orders can open additional opportunities and answers for the intricate difficulties presented via air contamination.

Value and civil rights should support natural strategies to guarantee that the weight of contamination doesn't excessively influence weak networks. Frequently, underestimated populaces endure the worst part of ecological corruption, living in regions with high contamination levels and restricted admittance to assets. Natural equity involves tending to these inconsistencies, guaranteeing that all networks have equivalent admittance to clean air, water, and a solid climate. Comprehensive strategies that consider the necessities and points of view of different networks add to an additional impartial and economical future.

The monetary area can go about as a strong impetus for change by incorporating ecological contemplations into speculation choices. Reasonable money, enveloping green securities, influence speculations, and moral financial practices, channels capital towards harmless to the ecosystem projects. Monetary establishments can use their impact to urge organizations with take on economical practices and comply to ecological guidelines. By adjusting monetary motivations to natural objectives, the monetary area turns into a main impetus in the change towards a cleaner, more economical worldwide economy.

Individual decisions and way of life changes are indispensable to the aggregate work to dispel any confusion. Straightforward activities, like decreasing energy utilization, limiting waste, and embracing eco-accommodating propensities, add to a more feasible lifestyle. The force of individual decisions stretches out to customer conduct, with reliable buying choices impacting market patterns. By embracing a practical ethos in day to day existence, people become problem solvers, on the whole guiding society towards an all the more naturally cognizant future.

## 9.1 Advocacy for tobacco control and public health policies

Tobacco use stays an inescapable worldwide general wellbeing challenge, adding to a heap of infections, financial weights, and unexpected losses. As the hindering wellbeing impacts of tobacco utilization become progressively apparent, the requirement for far reaching tobacco control measures and compelling general wellbeing strategies has never been more basic. Backing, established in proof based exploration and local area commitment, assumes an essential part in molding and carrying out strategies that relieve the effect of tobacco on people and social orders.

At the core of the backing for tobacco control is the acknowledgment of tobacco use as a main source of preventable sicknesses and demise around the world. Smoking, specifically, is a significant gamble factor for cardiovascular infections, respiratory problems, and different kinds of malignant growth.

Handed-down cigarette smoke, which influences non-smokers, represents extra wellbeing gambles, making tobacco a critical general wellbeing concern. The financial weight related with treating tobacco-related ailments further highlights the direness of carrying out strategies that check tobacco use.

Endeavors to control tobacco use are established in the affirmation of its habit-forming nature and the strategies utilized by the tobacco business to propagate its boundless utilization. Nicotine, the essential psychoactive part of tobacco, makes reliance, making it provoking for people to stop. Besides, forceful advertising techniques, especially focusing on weak populaces, add to the commencement and propagation of tobacco use. Support tries to neutralize these impacts by bringing issues to light, testing industry practices, and encouraging approaches that safeguard general wellbeing.

One of the foundations of tobacco control support is the advancement of proof based strategies. Thorough exploration and information investigation give the establishment to making powerful procedures to lessen tobacco use. This incorporates measures like tax assessment, sans smoke conditions, realistic admonition names, and complete tobacco promoting boycotts. Advocates work intimately with specialists, policymakers, and general wellbeing specialists to guarantee that approaches are grounded in logical proof and custom-made to the particular difficulties looked by different networks.

Tax collection, as a tobacco control procedure, has shown to be one of the best method for decreasing tobacco utilization. Higher tobacco costs deter inception and empower discontinuance, especially among youth and low-pay populaces. Advocates draw in with policymakers to carry out and increment tobacco charges, underscoring the potential for income age and the positive effect on general wellbeing results. In addition, income produced from tobacco assessments can be reserved for wellbeing advancement programs, further building up the connection between tax collection, general wellbeing, and local area prosperity.

Establishing sans smoke conditions addresses one more basic part of tobacco control promotion. Sans smoke approaches, which confine smoking openly places, work environments, and sporting facilities, add to lessening openness to handed-down cigarette smoke. Advocates work cooperatively with officials and local area pioneers to institute and fortify sans smoke regulation. By outlining without smoke arrangements as measures that safeguard the strength of non-smokers, including kids and pregnant ladies, advocates collect open help and establish conditions that advance better ways of life.

Realistic admonition marks on tobacco items act as an amazing asset for conveying the wellbeing chances related with smoking. Advocates champion the execution and improvement of realistic advance notice marks, stressing their adequacy in conveying the risks of tobacco use. Research demonstrates that such marks illuminate shoppers as well as hinder inception and empower discontinuance.

Through open mindfulness crusades, promotion endeavors expect to assemble support for strategies commanding conspicuous and effective admonition marks on all tobacco bundling.

Tobacco publicizing and advancement have for quite some time been distinguished as significant supporters of the predominance of tobacco use, particularly among youth. Advocates endeavor to check the impact of the tobacco business by advancing exhaustive prohibitions on tobacco publicizing, advancement, and sponsorship. This remembers limitations for customary promoting stations like TV, radio, and print media, as well as more current stages like virtual entertainment. By controlling the range and effect of tobacco promoting, backing tries to establish a climate that limits the appeal of tobacco items, especially among susceptible populaces.

Key to viable backing is the acknowledgment of the financial determinants of tobacco use. Weak populaces, incorporating those with lower financial status, are frequently lopsidedly impacted by tobacco-related sicknesses. Perceiving this, advocates work to tailor arrangements that address the interesting difficulties looked by these networks. This might include designated public mindfulness crusades, local area based mediations, and joint efforts with nearby associations to guarantee that tobacco control endeavors are comprehensive and address wellbeing differences.

Worldwide joint effort is a foundation of fruitful tobacco control promotion. Given the transnational idea of the tobacco business, collaboration between nations is fundamental to check cross-line showcasing and administrative escape clauses. Systems like the WHO Structure Show on Tobacco Control (FCTC) give a stage to countries to cooperate in creating and carrying out successful tobacco control strategies. Advocates assume a vital part in cultivating this joint effort, encouraging states to sanction and stick to peaceful accords that focus on general wellbeing over business interests.

Promotion reaches out past regulative measures to incorporate suit as a device to consider the tobacco business responsible for its activities. Legitimate activity against tobacco organizations has been instrumental in uncovering industry strategies, uncovering inward records, and getting pay for the wellbeing related costs brought about by states. Advocates team up with lawful specialists to assemble arguments against the tobacco business, utilizing the overall set of laws to uncover unfortunate behavior, look for equity for casualties, and beat unscrupulous practices down.

Local area commitment is a key part of successful backing for tobacco control. Engaging people group to take responsibility for wellbeing and prosperity includes bringing issues to light, giving assets to end, and encouraging a feeling of aggregate liability. Advocates work with local area pioneers, medical services suppliers, and instructors to foster socially delicate missions that reverberate with different populaces.

By intensifying the voices of those straightforwardly impacted by tobacco-related issues, support guarantees that arrangements are proof based as well as intelligent of the interesting requirements and points of view of various networks.

Youth commitment addresses a basic feature of tobacco control backing. Perceiving the defenselessness of youngsters to tobacco commencement, advocates put resources into instructive drives that furnish youth with the information and abilities to oppose tobacco use. School-based programs, shared missions, and drives utilizing virtual entertainment stages are utilized to reach and impact youth populaces. By encouraging a culture of sans tobacco living among the more youthful age, advocates mean to make a reasonable change in cultural standards and mentalities towards tobacco.

Neutralizing the tobacco business' endeavors to subvert general wellbeing approaches requires cautiousness and strength. Advocates intently screen industry exercises, uncovering misleading practices, and countering deception. By examining promoting methodologies, industry-supported research, and political campaigning, advocates expect to shield the respectability of general wellbeing arrangements. Besides, straightforwardness in communications between the tobacco business and policymakers is fundamental, and supporters work to guarantee that leaders focus on general wellbeing over corporate interests.

The job of medical services experts is crucial in tobacco control backing. Doctors, medical attendants, and other medical services suppliers act as believed wellsprings of data and backing for people trying to stop tobacco use. Advocates team up with medical care associations to incorporate tobacco discontinuance intercessions into clinical work on, guaranteeing that patients get exhaustive help. Furthermore, medical services experts assume an essential part in supporting for strategy changes, utilizing their skill to impact popular assessment and shape proof based approaches.

All in all, support for tobacco control and general wellbeing strategies is a diverse undertaking that requires joint effort across disciplines, areas, and networks. By utilizing proof based research, connecting with networks, and countering industry impact, advocates add to the turn of events and execution of strategies that safeguard people from the damages of tobacco use. A definitive objective isn't just to decrease the commonness of tobacco utilization however to establish conditions that cultivate better ways of life and focus on the prosperity of current and people in the future.

## 9.2 Innovative approaches to smoking cessation

Smoking suspension, the most common way of stopping tobacco use, is a perplexing excursion that includes both physiological and mental difficulties. With the deep rooted wellbeing chances related with smoking, including cardiovascular sicknesses, respiratory problems, and different diseases, tracking down viable and inventive ways to deal with assistance people quit smoking is of vital significance.

Conventional techniques, like advising and pharmacotherapy, have been basic in smoking end endeavors. Be that as it may, the scene is developing, and new, inventive methodologies are arising to address the different requirements and inclinations of those looking to stop smoking.

Advanced innovation has changed different parts of our lives, and smoking discontinuance is no special case. Portable applications, online stages, and wearable gadgets have become significant apparatuses in supporting people on their excursion to stop smoking. Smoking suspension applications offer customized plans, progress following, and inspirational messages to clients. These applications influence conduct science standards, giving ongoing criticism and backing that lines up with a person's stopped arrangement. Some applications even integrate gamification components, transforming the discontinuance cycle into a seriously captivating and intelligent experience.

Wearable gadgets, for example, smartwatches and wellness trackers, add to smoking end by checking actual work, pulse, and even feelings of anxiety. These gadgets give clients an all encompassing perspective on their wellbeing and prosperity, building up the positive effect of stopping smoking. Also, a few wearable innovations offer elements like customized instructing and warnings to urge clients to remain without smoke. The reconciliation of advanced apparatuses into smoking discontinuance programs improves openness as well as considers persistent, constant help, tending to the powerful idea of the stopping system.

Computer generated reality (VR) addresses a creative outskirts in smoking discontinuance mediations. VR innovation drenches people in recreated conditions, giving an exceptional stage to remedial mediations. Computer generated reality treatment for smoking end includes presenting people to situations that trigger desires in a controlled and strong setting. This openness treatment, joined with mental social methods, assists people with creating survival techniques and desensitize their reactions to smoking signals. VR mediations offer a protected and controlled space for rehearsing refusal abilities, making it a promising road for upgrading customary conduct treatments.

Telehealth has acquired unmistakable quality as a helpful and open method for conveying smoking end mediations. Remote directing meetings, either through video calls or phone discussions, interface people with prepared experts who give direction and backing. Telehealth kills geological hindrances, permitting people to get to guiding administrations from the solace of their homes. Also, it takes special care of different populaces, remembering those for provincial or underserved regions, who might confront difficulties in getting to face to face suspension administrations. The adaptability of telehealth administrations obliges occupied plans and fluctuating inclinations, making it an inventive and comprehensive way to deal with smoking end.

Care and reflection have found a spot in smoking end programs, offering people a comprehensive way to deal with overseeing desires and stress. Care rehearses, like careful breathing and contemplation, develop familiarity with the current second, assisting people with breaking the programmed and constant nature of smoking. Care based smoking discontinuance programs incorporate these practices with mental conduct methodologies, giving an exhaustive tool compartment to people to explore the difficulties of stopping. By encouraging a careful consciousness of triggers and reactions, people can foster a more noteworthy feeling of command over their smoking way of behaving.

Pharmacogenetics, the investigation of how hereditary variables impact a singular's reaction to drugs, is preparing for customized smoking discontinuance medicines. Hereditary varieties can affect how the body utilizes prescriptions utilized in smoking suspension, impacting their adequacy and expected aftereffects. Pharmacogenetic testing permits medical services suppliers to fit discontinuance drugs to a person's hereditary profile, advancing therapy results. This customized approach holds guarantee for working on quit rates and limiting unfriendly responses, addressing a stage towards accuracy medication in smoking end.

Virtual entertainment stages have become amazing assets for making steady networks and encouraging companion associations among people endeavoring to stop smoking. Online gatherings, gatherings, and virtual entertainment crusades give spaces to people to share their encounters, offer help, and celebrate achievements. The feeling of local area and shared obligation to stopping improves inspiration and responsibility. Furthermore, web-based entertainment stages can be used for designated smoking suspension crusades, contacting assorted crowds and scattering proof based data.

Message informing intercessions, otherwise called SMS-based mediations, profit by the omnipresence of cell phones to convey opportune and customized help for smoking suspension. Robotized instant messages can give persuasive substance, survival techniques, and updates for prescription adherence. The nonconcurrent idea of text informing obliges individual inclinations and encourages a feeling of independence in the stopping system. Research demonstrates that text informing mediations can essentially work on quit rates, making them a savvy and versatile way to deal with smoking suspension support.

Man-made consciousness (artificial intelligence) is progressively being coordinated into smoking discontinuance mediations, offering customized and versatile help. Man-made intelligence calculations dissect client information, including smoking examples, triggers, and profound states, to fit intercessions to individual requirements. Chatbots controlled by computer based intelligence draw in with clients continuously, offering moment help, consolation, and survival techniques. The consistent learning capacity of simulated intelligence permits mediations to develop in light of client criticism and results, making a dynamic and responsive framework for smoking suspension support.

Monetary impetuses and rewards present a creative way to deal with inspire people to stop smoking. Monetary motivation programs offer money related rewards or limits for people who effectively quit smoking or take part in smoking end exercises. The possibility of substantial prizes gives an extra layer of inspiration, tending to the monetary part of smoking suspension. These projects can be carried out in working environment settings, medical services frameworks, or local area drives, making an uplifting feedback component to energize and support smoking restraint.

Peer support, worked with through bunch guiding or shared help associations, stays a strong and creative system in smoking end. The feeling of local area and divided encounters between people pursuing the shared objective of stopping smoking encourages a strong climate. Peer support programs give a stage to people to trade ways of dealing with hardship or stress, celebrate victories, and explore difficulties together. This relational association upgrades inspiration and versatility, adding to the general progress of smoking discontinuance endeavors.

Biomedical intercessions, for example, immunizations focusing on nicotine, address a state of the art way to deal with smoking discontinuance. Nicotine immunizations animate the resistant framework to deliver antibodies that tight spot to nicotine atoms, keeping them from arriving at the mind and evoking the compensating impacts related with smoking. While still in the trial stage, these immunizations hold guarantee as long haul smoking discontinuance helps. By decreasing the building up properties of nicotine, immunizations could assist people with stopping smoking and forestall backslide, offering a novel and possibly game-changing road for intercession.

Natural intercessions influence the physical and social climate to make conditions that help smoking end. This incorporates arrangements and drives that advance without smoke spaces, confine tobacco publicizing, and denormalize smoking in group environments. Clean air regulations, which preclude smoking out in the open spots, add to changing normal practices and decreasing the perceivability of smoking. Such natural changes supplement individual-level mediations, making an exhaustive methodology that tends to both the miniature and full scale impacts on smoking way of behaving.

Mix of smoking end into essential consideration settings addresses a shift towards a comprehensive and patient-focused approach. By installing end administrations inside routine medical care visits, people get ceaseless help and direction from their medical services suppliers. This approach gains by the trust and compatibility among patients and medical care experts, making it more probable for people to look for and stick to smoking suspension mediations. Coordinating discontinuance support into essential consideration guarantees that stopping smoking is drawn closer as a key part of generally wellbeing and prosperity.

Social ability in smoking end mediations recognizes the variety of people and fits ways to deal with explicit social settings. Socially delicate projects think about semantic, social, and social factors that impact smoking way of behaving and stopping inclinations. This includes working together with local area pioneers, integrating social images and practices into intercessions, and perceiving the one of a kind difficulties looked by changed ethnic and social gatherings. By regarding and embracing variety, social skill improves the pertinence and viability of smoking.

### 9.3 The potential for a smoke-free future and the role of society in achieving it

The vision of a sans smoke future is a strong and groundbreaking yearning that rises above individual wellbeing and reaches out to the prosperity of social orders all in all. It imagines a reality where the hurtful effects of tobacco use are limited, and networks flourish in a climate liberated from the weights of smoking-related sicknesses. Understanding this vision requires a deliberate exertion from all areas of society, enveloping states, medical services frameworks, networks, organizations, and people. The excursion towards a without smoke future isn't just a general wellbeing basic however a cultural obligation that requests joint effort, development, and supported responsibility.

Integral to the quest for a sans smoke future is the acknowledgment of the staggering wellbeing outcomes related with tobacco use. Smoking remaining parts a main source of preventable illnesses, adding to cardiovascular infections, respiratory problems, and different types of malignant growth. The financial weight of treating tobacco-related sicknesses overwhelms medical care frameworks and blocks social and monetary turn of events. As social orders take a stab at better and stronger networks, tending to the underlying drivers of tobacco-related illnesses becomes principal.

States assume a urgent part in forming the direction towards a sans smoke future. The execution of proof based tobacco control strategies is a foundation of general wellbeing endeavors. Complete tobacco control measures incorporate tobacco tax assessment, without smoke approaches, realistic admonition names, promoting limitations, and admittance to smoking end administrations. States should sanction and authorize these arrangements to establish a climate that deters tobacco use and supports people in their excursion to stop. The obligation to strong tobacco control strategies mirrors a general public's devotion to focusing on the wellbeing and prosperity of its residents.

Tax collection stands apart as an amazing asset in decreasing tobacco utilization and supporting general wellbeing drives. Higher tobacco costs put commencement among youth as well down as propel current smokers to stop. Income created from tobacco assessments can be reserved for wellbeing advancement programs, further supporting the association between tobacco tax collection and cultural prosperity. Legislatures should oppose industry pressures and focus on general wellbeing over financial contemplations while planning and changing tobacco charge arrangements.

Sans smoke approaches, which limit smoking openly places, working environments, and sporting facilities, add to establishing conditions that help smoking discontinuance and safeguard non-smokers from handed-down cigarette smoke. States should take on and implement solid without smoke regulation, perceiving that these strategies add to a culture shift towards a sans smoke standard. By denormalizing smoking openly spaces, social orders send an unmistakable message about the inadmissibility of tobacco use and prepare for a future where smoking is an undeniably interesting and socially beat conduct down.

Realistic admonition names on tobacco items are instrumental in imparting the wellbeing chances related with smoking. State run administrations ought to order unmistakable and significant admonition names, guaranteeing that buyers are very much educated about the perils regarding tobacco use. These marks act as a hindrance as well as add to public mindfulness and schooling. Cultural help for realistic advance notice names mirrors an aggregate obligation to engaging people with the data they need to pursue informed decisions about their wellbeing.

Promoting limitations address a pivotal part of tobacco control, as the tobacco business has a past filled with utilizing modern showcasing methodologies to target weak populaces, particularly youth. State run administrations should execute thorough restrictions on tobacco publicizing, advancement, and sponsorship across different media channels, including customary outlets and arising computerized stages. By destroying the limited time apparatus of the tobacco business, social orders can shield general wellbeing and forestall the enrollment of new smokers.

Admittance to smoking discontinuance administrations is a central part of a complete tobacco control system. Legislatures ought to put resources into and advance the accessibility of proof based end programs, guaranteeing that people have the help they need to stop smoking. This incorporates advising administrations, pharmacotherapy, and imaginative computerized mediations that take care of different inclinations and necessities. The coordination of smoking discontinuance administrations into essential medical services settings upgrades openness and supports the thought that stopping smoking is an indispensable piece of in general wellbeing and prosperity.

Medical services frameworks bear a common obligation in the excursion towards a without smoke future. Past giving suspension administrations, medical care experts should effectively take part in tobacco control endeavors through routine screening, advising, and training. Incorporating tobacco discontinuance support into routine clinical consideration guarantees that each medical services experience turns into a valuable chance to address smoking way of behaving. Besides, medical care experts act as persuasive backers for tobacco control approaches, utilizing their skill to shape general assessment and energize strategy changes.

Local area commitment is basic in encouraging a cultural obligation to a sans smoke future. Nearby associations, grassroots developments, and local area pioneers assume a crucial part in preparing support for tobacco control drives. Local area based mediations, instructive projects, and mindfulness crusades add to changing accepted practices and mentalities towards smoking. By establishing conditions that help stopping and advance without smoke living, networks become impetuses for more extensive cultural change.

Organizations, both enormous companies and little endeavors, play a part to play in propelling a without smoke future. Executing without smoke working environment arrangements safeguards the soundness of representatives as well as adds to the standardization of sans smoke conditions. Bosses can uphold smoking discontinuance endeavors by giving assets, guiding administrations, and motivators for workers trying to stop. Past the working environment, organizations can add to a sans smoke future by taking on dependable showcasing rehearses and shunning organizations with the tobacco business.

The media, as a strong force to be reckoned with of general assessment, assumes a significant part in forming cultural perspectives towards smoking. News sources ought to effectively take part in enemy of smoking efforts, disperse proof based data about the wellbeing dangers of tobacco use, and check supportive of tobacco messages. By utilizing their range and impact, the media can add to building public mindfulness and encouraging a cultural story that rejects smoking as a standard.

Instructive establishments have an interesting an open door to shape the perspectives and ways of behaving of people in the future. Coordinating complete tobacco instruction into school educational plans outfits understudies with the information and abilities to settle on informed conclusions about tobacco use. Counteraction programs, peer-drove drives, and instructive missions add to making an age that sees tobacco use as incongruent with a sound and fruitful life. Instructive organizations become key accomplices in developing a sans tobacco outlook since the beginning.

Non-legislative associations (NGOs) and promotion bunches assume an essential part in considering legislatures and organizations responsible for their responsibilities to tobacco control. These associations give a stage to grassroots activism, participate in open mindfulness missions, and hall for strategy changes. Their part in preparing public help, bringing issues to light about the tobacco business' strategies, and pushing for more grounded guidelines is fundamental in balancing the impact of strong tobacco organizations.

People, as citizenry, have a moral obligation in adding to a without smoke future. Stopping smoking is an individual excursion, and people should effectively search out and use accessible suspension assets. Support from loved ones, cooperation in local area based end projects, and commitment with computerized apparatuses can upgrade a singular's opportunities to effectively stop.

By getting a sense of ownership with their wellbeing and effectively partaking in tobacco control endeavors, people become problem solvers in the more extensive cultural development towards a sans smoke future.

Development and examination are essential parts of the excursion towards a without smoke future. Putting resources into research on compelling end mediations, novel advancements, and arising patterns in tobacco use permits social orders to remain on top of things. Advancement in smoking end treatments, like the improvement of new meds or the refinement of existing methodologies, adds to growing the tool stash accessible to people looking to stop. In addition, research on the developing scene of tobacco items, including arising nicotine conveyance frameworks, illuminates approaches that address new difficulties in tobacco control.

Worldwide cooperation is fundamental in tending to the worldwide idea of the tobacco plague. The World Wellbeing Association (WHO) Structure Show on Tobacco Control (FCTC) fills in as a directing system for worldwide tobacco control endeavors. Nations should team up to share best practices, trade data, and aggregately address cross-line difficulties presented by the tobacco business. Global organizations improve the aggregate effect of individual countries, cultivating a common obligation to making a smoke-liberated world.

Accomplishing a without smoke future isn't simply an errand for legislatures or medical care frameworks alone; it requires the dynamic and aggregate support of society all in all. Society assumes a vital part in forming the standards, mentalities, and ways of behaving that impact tobacco use. From people and families to networks, organizations, instructive foundations, and non-legislative associations, each section of society adds to the more extensive exertion of establishing a climate where smoking is deterred, wellbeing is focused on, and the weight of tobacco-related illnesses is essentially diminished.

At the center of society's job in accomplishing a without smoke future is the development of mindfulness and training. Information is an amazing asset in the battle against tobacco use, and society should effectively take part in dispersing data about the wellbeing gambles related with smoking. Instructive missions, both at the local area and public levels, can assist with bringing issues to light about the risks of tobacco, the advantages of stopping, and the assets accessible for those trying to stop. A very much educated society is better prepared to settle on sound decisions and add to a social shift away from tobacco use.

Families, as the essential unit of society, apply a significant effect on people's mentalities towards smoking. Guardians, kin, and more distant family individuals assume vital parts in molding the early impression of tobacco use. Establishing a sans smoke home climate shields relatives from handed-down cigarette smoke as well as sets a strong model for kids.

Guardians, specifically, act as good examples, and their perspectives towards smoking essentially influence the smoking way of behaving of their kids. Family-based intercessions that advance open correspondence about the dangers of smoking and offer help for stopping add to building an establishment for a without smoke future.

Networks, enveloping areas, nearby associations, and grassroots developments, are fundamental in encouraging a strong climate for smoking suspension. Local area drove drives, for example, without smoke crusades, neighborhood support gatherings, and mindfulness programs, add to switching normal practices up tobacco use. By making spaces where smoking is deterred, networks effectively shape the view of smoking as a bothersome way of behaving. In addition, local area commitment is crucial in pushing for and supporting nearby approaches that advance without smoke living, for example, clean air statutes and limitations on tobacco promoting.

Organizations assume a double part in the excursion towards a without smoke future. On one hand, organizations can add to a sans smoke climate by embracing and upholding sans smoke working environment strategies. Past lawful necessities, businesses can execute smoking discontinuance programs, give assets to representatives looking to stop, and make a culture that upholds wellbeing and prosperity. Then again, organizations should be cautious about their practices and keep away from associations with the tobacco business. Corporate obligation reaches out to avoiding publicizing tobacco items and effectively adding to tobacco control endeavors inside the networks they work.

Instructive foundations employ huge impact in molding the discernments and ways of behaving of people in the future. By coordinating far reaching tobacco instruction into school educational programs, instructive foundations add to building an age that is very much educated about the dangers regarding smoking. Counteraction programs, peer-drove drives, and hostile to smoking efforts inside schools assume a significant part in making a culture that rejects tobacco use. Past proper schooling, colleges and universities can execute without smoke grounds strategies, further supporting the message that training and a sound way of life remain closely connected.

Non-Administrative Associations (NGOs) and backing bunches are instrumental in activating society and considering partners responsible for their responsibilities to tobacco control. NGOs give a stage to grassroots activism, participate in open mindfulness missions, and hall for strategy changes. Their part in teaching people in general about the strategies of the tobacco business, pushing for more grounded guidelines, and supporting people trying to stop is basic. NGOs go about as guard dogs, guaranteeing that the voice of the general population is heard, and that approaches focus on general wellbeing over business interests.

People, as citizenry, are key problem solvers in the mission for a without smoke future. Stopping smoking is an individual excursion, and people should effectively search out and use accessible suspension assets.

Support from loved ones, cooperation in local area based discontinuance projects, and commitment with advanced devices can improve a singular's opportunities to effectively stop. Moral obligation regarding one's wellbeing stretches out past stopping smoking to pushing for and supporting tobacco control endeavors in the more extensive local area. People should perceive their job in molding cultural standards and effectively partake in the development towards a sans smoke future.

Development and exploration are essential parts of society's commitment to accomplishing a without smoke future. Research on viable discontinuance mediations, arising patterns in tobacco use, and the effect of arrangements assists social orders with remaining on the ball. Advancement in smoking suspension treatments, like the improvement of new meds or the refinement of existing methodologies, adds to growing the tool stash accessible to people looking to stop. Additionally, research on the developing scene of tobacco items, including arising nicotine conveyance frameworks, illuminates arrangements that address new difficulties in tobacco control.

News sources, as strong forces to be reckoned with of popular assessment, assume an essential part in molding cultural perspectives towards smoking. The media can contribute essentially to building public mindfulness and cultivating a cultural story that rejects smoking as a standard. By scattering proof based data about the wellbeing dangers of tobacco use, countering supportive of tobacco messages, and taking part in enemy of smoking efforts, news sources influence their range and impact for the more noteworthy public great. Dependable covering tobacco-related issues adds to making an educated and drew in the public eye.

States, as delegates of society's aggregate will, are key designers of strategies that shape the climate towards a sans smoke future. Execution and authorization of proof based tobacco control approaches are pivotal moves toward establishing a climate that deters tobacco use. Legislatures should oppose industry pressures and focus on general wellbeing over financial contemplations while forming and changing tobacco control approaches. Through regulation, guideline, and general wellbeing drives, legislatures mirror the qualities and needs of the social orders they address.

Worldwide coordinated effort is crucial in tending to the worldwide idea of the tobacco plague. The World Wellbeing Association (WHO) Structure Show on Tobacco Control (FCTC) fills in as a directing system for worldwide tobacco control endeavors. Nations should team up to share best practices, trade data, and altogether address cross-line difficulties presented by the tobacco business. Global organizations upgrade the aggregate effect of individual countries, encouraging a common obligation to making a smoke-liberated world.

www.ingramcontent.com/pod-product-compliance
Lightning Source LLC
LaVergne TN
LVHW021828060526
838201LV00058B/3558